ROSE REISMAN'S
CHOOSE IT
AND LOSE IT

ROSE REISMAN'S

CHOOSE IT
AND LOSE IT

**The road map
to healthier
eating at your
favourite Canadian
restaurants**

whitecap

PUBLISHER: Michael Burch
EDITING: Lara Kordić
DESIGN: Mauve Pagé (mauvepage.com)
FOOD PHOTOGRAPHY & STYLING: Mike McColl

PRINTED IN CANADA

Library and Archives Canada Cataloguing in Publication

Rose Reisman's choose it and lose it : the road map to healthier eating at your favourite Canadian restaurants.

Includes index.

ISBN 978-1-77050-099-0

1. Restaurants. 2. Convenience foods— Health aspects. 3. Nutrition. I. Title. II. Title: Choose It and Lose It

RA784.R457 2012   613.2   C2011-908307-8

The publisher acknowledges the financial support of the Government of Canada through the Canada Book Fund (CBF) and the Province of British Columbia through the Book Publishing Tax Credit.

12 13 14 15 16   5 4 3 2 1

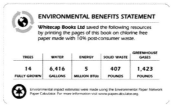

ENVIRONMENTAL BENEFITS STATEMENT

Whitecap Books Ltd saved the following resources by printing the pages of this book on chlorine free paper made with 10% post-consumer waste.

TREES	WATER	ENERGY	SOLID WASTE	GREENHOUSE GASES
14	6,416	5	407	1,423
FULLY GROWN	GALLONS	MILLION BTUs	POUNDS	POUNDS

Environmental impact estimates were made using the Environmental Paper Network Paper Calculator. For more information visit www.papercalculator.org.

The nutritional information given for the restaurant meals in this book was obtained directly from each restaurant, either online or on site, and was correct as of June 2012.

DEDICATION

My drive and energy for each day comes from my incredible family. I began my career when I was a mother of four young children. As my children have all left the nest I have been able to give more time to my work, for which I live and breathe, on a daily basis.

Natalie Reisman Breger – She's now married and a lawyer. How lucky can a mother be! Ricky, her husband, is the best son-in-law one could hope for.

David Reisman – My wonderful, bright and so good-looking son. You have a smile that lights up a room.

Laura Reisman – A warm, sensitive and incredible young woman. I love your passion for your work and life.

Adam Reisman – Always the baby. Finding his way and exploring his independence.

Sam Reisman – My true inspiration and love of my life. No one has loved me more.

My animal clan of two German Shephards and two cats. The serenity at night as they all sleep on my bed despite the wishes of my husband.

My two best buddies, Kathy Kacer and Susan Gordin, with whom I share my life.

CONTENTS

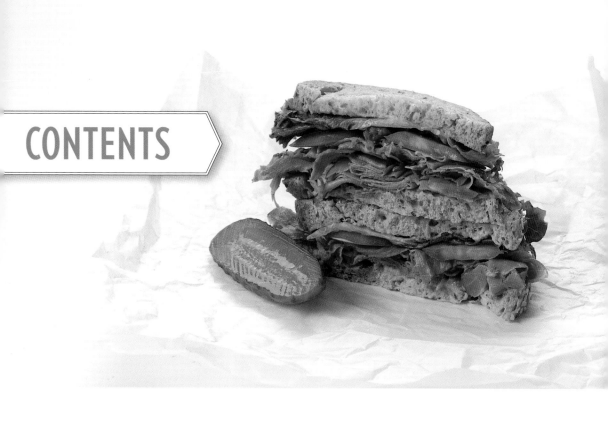

FOREWORD

What if you could add 7.5 years to your life—years in which you would be largely healthy and able to participate freely in life activities?

The key to making this a reality is outlined in a recent study by the Institute of Clinical Evaluative Studies (ICES) and the Public Health Agency of Canada that took place in Ontario in April 2012, which found you can achieve a substantial increase in your life expectancy and quality of life by following these five habits:

» being physically active
» eating healthy, nutritious food
» not smoking
» drinking alcohol in moderation (if you do drink)
» managing stress.

There was a dramatic difference between those individuals who followed none of these healthy habits and those who followed all five. For men, the difference ranged from 68.5 years to 88.6 years, and for women it ranged from 71.5 years to 92.5 years. More good news: those who followed the habits had fewer chronic conditions and disabilities, which are major health concerns as we age. Social, economic and physical conditions are also very important. People living in Ontario's poorest communities have a life expectancy that is 4.5 years less than those in wealthier communities.

In the Faculty of Health at York University, one of our goals is to keep "more people healthier longer." This can best be accomplished by initiatives that enable people to follow these five healthy habits and by addressing social conditions that can make healthier choices easier, especially in poorer communities.

Without doubt, one of the most difficult habits to adopt is to eat healthy, nutritious food. Every day, we have to make decisions regarding what we eat. The choices between healthier and less healthy food can be quite perplexing, especially in restaurants, where many of us are eating more and more often.

This is where my colleague Rose Reisman, an adjunct professor in the faculty, has done a remarkable service, with her latest book *Rose Reisman's Choose it and Lose it*. This book will help you make better choices when you are eating out at restaurants. Rose provides us with a simple way to navigate a myriad of menu options. This very practical book is an invaluable tool that can help Canadians achieve healthier lifestyles.

—Harvey Skinner, PhD
Dean, Faculty of Health, York University, Toronto
Fellow of the Canadian Academy of Health Sciences
Certified Psychologist

WHY I WROTE THIS BOOK

If you've just picked up this book (my 17th) expecting to find a new set of delicious light cooking ideas, you are probably surprised to see that this time I've decided to take a different approach. By now you know how to eat and cook in a healthy way at home, but you may not know how to apply the good habits you have when eating in restaurants.

How can you determine which menu items are the healthiest? You could order a salad or go for the vegetarian option, but those are not always safe bets. For instance, who would have thought that Manchu Wok's Honey Garlic Chicken has 450 calories with 22 grams of fat, while its Black Pepper Chicken has 160 calories, with 10 grams of fat What about McDonald's Bacon and Egg Bagel? It has 530 calories and 26 grams of fat, compared with the Egg McMuffin, which has a mere 290 calories and 12 grams of fat. As you will learn in *Choose It and Lose It,* just because it looks like a duck and walks like duck, doesn't mean it's a duck. Foods that sound healthy aren't necessarily the best option for you.

This book would not be necessary if restaurants were more open about what goes in their food. Consumers should not have to dive deep into a corporate website to study the nutritional information for menu items or ask for a nutrient brochure that reads like a set of mathematical equations. I believe that nutritional values should appear on a menu, complete with a contextual guide. However, until they do, you have *Choose It and Lose It* to help you navigate your way through fast food and chain restaurant menus.

Every day in the news we are bombarded with information and advice about healthy living. We can find out the nutrients in every item in our grocery store shopping cart by looking at the package or we can go online and read about the ingredients in our favourite restaurant dishes. We're regularly warned about the amount of money that goes into our nation's health budget. Patients with diseases and health concerns such as obesity, type 2 diabetes, heart disease and certain cancers are now taking up 70 percent of the space in our hospitals. Although we know that the prevalence of these conditions could be significantly reduced if we ate better and adopted healthier lifestyles, our health as a nation is not improving. All the preaching about achieving a healthier population has fallen on deaf ears. Knowing that excess sodium can lead to high blood pressure, that saturated fat clogs our arteries, that smoked meats have been linked to stomach and colon cancer and that obesity leads to type 2 diabetes hasn't changed our daily eating habits.

But what if I were to show you how you can eat in any restaurant or fast-food spot in Canada and always make a better choice while avoiding thousands of calories. You would lose weight without ever going on another diet! You can still enjoy a burger or donut, but the burger or donut that is healthier, one that can eventually make a difference in your weight and health over time.

The typical Canadian eats out 11 times during a two-week period. We need to recognize that fast-food restaurants and chains account for a good deal of our society's health issues. The *Montreal Gazette* recently reported that nutrition-related diseases, including stroke, diabetes, heart disease and certain cancers, kill an estimated 48,000 Canadians every year and cost about $7 billion in health care. But we can turn this terrible statistic around. If we don't, we run the risk of consuming our national budgets on health expenditures as we live shorter and profoundly less satisfying lives. Changing our eating habits is imperative. But until the restaurant industry reaches a reasonable standard of self-regulation and addresses increased consumer and government demand for greater transparency and healthier options, the burden falls on us to educate ourselves. This is why *Choose It and Lose It* is an indispensable resource for informing and changing consumers' eating habits.

Choose It and Lose It will surprise and at times upset you as you learn the truths and the trade-offs that are behind so many popular menu items. The good news is that you can change things simply by making more informed decisions while eating out. The information in this book is easy to access, and by following just some of the book's recommendations you can shed literally tens of pounds a year!

I have been criticized for recommending fast-food and chain restaurant menu items. In response, I say the only way we are going to win the battle against obesity and disease is to make small, gradual changes. The alternative would be a book called *Don't Eat Here, or Here, or Here,* which wouldn't be very constructive. Denying that the fast-food industry exists and has a profound impact on our health is like burying our heads in the sand. I believe that if consumers are equipped with relevant information, over time we will start to bypass high-calorie, high-fat and low-nutrition items in favour of healthier choices. In turn, the restaurant industry will respond by providing healthier items and eventually eliminate the very worst items from their menus. I hope this book will give you the steps you need to start leading a healthier life, one menu at a time.

Enjoy!

ROSE REISMAN

OUR CURRENT HEALTH CRISIS

Today's most prevalent health concerns, such as obesity, heart disease, type 2 diabetes and certain cancers, lead to shortened life expectancy and lower quality of life. A common factor in the development of these life-threatening conditions is the food we eat every day—namely, foods with excess calories, fat, sodium and sugar.

In 2010, an average of 39 percent of Canada's provincial budgets was spent on health care. Ontario and Manitoba spent the highest proportion of their budgets on health in 2009 (45.7 percent and 43.7 percent, respectively) while Newfoundland and Labrador and Quebec spent the lowest (33.8 percent and 33.1 percent, respectively).[01] With chronic disease on the increase, a greater and greater percentage of our provincial budgets will be devoted to health care in the coming years, and soon we will have a system that is ready to implode.

OBESITY—A NATIONAL EPIDEMIC

Canada, like many nations, is in the midst of an obesity epidemic, which is believed to be caused by an increase in calorie consumption over the past 20 years. Currently, 59 percent of adult Canadians are either overweight or obese. Table 1 shows obesity rates in each province in 2005.

Table 2 shows the average daily caloric intake per person in Canada from 1990 to 2007. In the past 15 years we have increased our daily caloric intake by an average of 500 calories. Individuals who add 500 calories to their diets every day, would gain 52 lb (24 kg) by the end of one year!

According to the Centre for Disease Control and Prevention, obesity is an abnormal accumulation of body fat, usually 20 percent or more over an individual's ideal body weight. For example, if a woman who is 5 feet 4 inches (162.5 centimetres) tall has an ideal body weight of 135 pounds (61 kilograms) but instead weighs over 160 pounds (73 kilograms), she is considered obese.

---

01   Canadian Institute for Health Information.
     http://www.cihi.ca

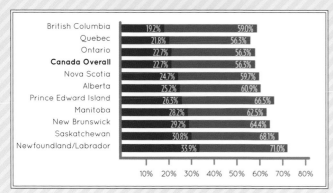

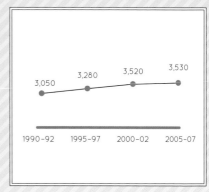

TABLE 1: Obesity Rates in Canadian Provinces in 2005 (*Note:* blue = percentage of population that is obese; red = percentage of population that is obese or overweight) *Source: Margot Shields and Michael Tjepkema. Statistics Canada. http://www.statcan.gc.ca/pub/82-003-x/2005003/article/9280-eng.pdf*

TABLE 2: Average Daily Caloric Intake per Capita in Canada from 1990 to 2007

After smoking, obesity is the second most preventable cause of death in North America.[02] There are many reasons for the increase in obesity, mainly inactivity, lack of food portion control and the proliferation of fast-food restaurants worldwide. About two out of three North Americans, including one in four children and adolescents, are considered overweight or obese.[03]

Obesity puts people at greater risk for developing chronic diseases. A significant percent of all deaths in Canada may be attributed to obesity. Obesity contributes to the development of the following conditions:

» coronary heart disease and stroke
» type 2 diabetes
» cancers: esophageal, breast (post-menopausal), endometrial, colorectal, kidney, pancreatic, thyroid, gall bladder and possibly other types[04]
» hypertension

» high cholesterol and high levels of triglycerides
» liver and gall bladder disease
» sleep apnea and respiratory problems
» osteoarthritis (degeneration of cartilage and its underlying bone within a joint)
» gynaecological problems (abnormal menses, infertility)

What is even worse is that 70 percent of kids who are overweight will be overweight adults, and 80 percent of overweight kids who have one overweight parent will continue to be overweight into adulthood. Obesity rates in children have almost tripled in the past 25 years. Approximately 26 percent of Canadian children are currently overweight or obese. Among teen boys between the ages of 15 and 19, the proportion classified as overweight or obese rose from 14 percent to 31 percent between 1981 and 2009. Among girls in the same age group, obesity rates rose from 14 percent to 25 percent.[05]

Today's children have life expectancies two to five years shorter than their parents'. They are now

02 World Health Organization. http://www.who.int/healthinfo/global_burden_disease/risk_factors/en/index.html
03 Nutrition in Clinical Practice. http://ncp.sagepub.com/content/26/5/510.extract
04 National Cancer Institute. http://cancer.gov/cancertopics/factsheet/Risk/obesity
05 Child Obesity Foundation. http://www.childhoodobesityfoundation.ca/statistics

developing "adult" diseases, such as type 2 diabetes, heart disease and cancer—not to mention depression and emotional and self-esteem issues that surface as a result of obesity. A study by the American Health Association reported children as young as 10 having prematurely aged neck arteries (that look like those of a 45-year-old), which puts them at risk for future heart disease and high cholesterol in their 20s and 30s.

When children eat out, like adults they consume more calories, fat, sodium and sugar than they would if they ate only home-cooked meals. Most restaurants want to create the largest portions using the least amount of money. The lowest cost comes from inexpensive ingredients, such as starch, sugar, salt and grease. That's why a Wendy's burger costs a lot less than a bowl of strawberries! Restaurants provide one-quarter of our children's meals but these meals add up to over one-third of our children's daily calories. Children's consumption of fast food has increased fivefold since the 1970s.

Where do our extra calories come from?

» High fructose corn syrup—this is an inexpensive ingredient used to replace sugar and other sweeteners. Fructose doesn't trigger hormone responses that regulate appetite and satiety, so it tricks you into overeating, causes weight gain and can lead to type 2 diabetes.
» Saturated fats and trans-fats—these taste great and are less expensive than healthy mono-unsaturated oils. These bad fats increase bad cholesterol (LDL), lower good cholesterol (HDL) and increase the risk of heart disease.
» Oil, mayonnaise, corn and soy fillers—these contain excess Omega-6 fatty acids, which lead to excess fat cells. Omega-6, like Omega-3 fatty acids, are an essential source of energy that is found in animal and vegetable fats and oils. But excess Omega-6 can lead to types 2 diabetes and heart disease. Our ratio of Omega-6 to Omega-3

fatty acids should be 1:1, but our average consumption is 20:1!
» Drinks—we are drinking our calories (as much as an extra 450 calories daily) in the form of pop, juices, coffee beverages, smoothies and milkshakes.
» "Supersizing" (ordering the largest size of a meal)—this might save us a few dollars in the short term, but it won't save our health in the long term.

DIABETES

This serious illness is now affecting both older and younger generations at an alarming pace. It is three times more common today than it was four decades ago, mostly due to increased obesity rates.

Diabetes is a condition in which the body either lacks insulin or cannot use it properly. Over 90 percent of diabetics suffer from the type 2 form of the disease. It is the seventh leading cause of death in North America and can lead to other serious health complications, including heart disease, blindness, kidney failure and lower-extremity amputations. Type 2 diabetes may shorten one's life expectancy by 5 to 10 years. A large proportion of cases are caused by obesity, genetics, high blood pressure and high blood cholesterol.[06] Being of Aboriginal, Hispanic, Asian, South Asian or South African descent may also increase one's risk of developing type 2 diabetes.

More than 20 people around the world are diagnosed with diabetes every hour. Between 2010 and 2020, another 1.2 million Canadians will be diagnosed with diabetes, bringing the total number of Canadians living with diabetes to 3.7 million—or 9.9 per cent of the population. In 2000, 4.2 percent of Canadians were living with the disease.[07] A child born in 2000 has a one in three chance of being diagnosed

---

06   Canadian Diabetes Association. Obesity. http://www.diabetes
      .ca/research/obesity/
07   Public Health Agency of Canada.

with type 2 diabetes in his or her lifetime.[08] However, losing even modest amounts of weight and getting more physical exercise may decrease one's blood sugar levels by as much as 60 percent and help prevent diabetes.

CANCER

What we eat affects our chances of developing certain cancers. Reducing obesity by limiting the saturated fats, hydrogenated fats, sodium and alcohol in our diets may reduce the incidence of specific cancers, as can increased activity. Up to 35 percent of all cancers can be prevented by being active, eating well and maintaining a healthy body weight.[09]

HEART DISEASE

Heart disease and stroke are two of the three leading causes of death in Canada, costing the Canadian economy more than $20.9 billion every year in physician services, hospital costs, lost wages and decreased productivity.[10] Cardiovascular diseases account for close to one-third of all Canadian deaths.

I know too many people who have died from a massive coronary before they reached the hospital. My father was one of these. He died in his mid-50s. He had all the risk factors for heart disease, including obesity, high cholesterol, high blood pressure and inactivity. For those lucky enough to survive a heart attack, a change in lifestyle can dramatically improve the chances of living a long and healthy life.

DAILY NUTRIENT REQUIREMENTS FOR OPTIMAL HEALTH

There are many different recommendations available for required daily nutrients. Many do not distinguish between an active or sedentary lifestyle. With the assistance of the Center for Food Safety and Applied Nutrition I have developed tables for both lifestyles (see page 08).

Women with active lifestyles who are over 50 have different nutrition requirements than women with active lifestyles who are aged 24 to 50 because of the effects of menopause (see Table 3A on page 08). These are only general recommendations and do not account for variations between individuals' metabolic rates. The more active your lifestyle, the more calories you can consume without gaining weight. All the recommendations in the restaurant listings are based on optimal nutrients for women with sedentary lifestyles (see Table 3B on page 08).

Following the recommended daily nutritional values may lead to a healthier body weight and even a healthier lifestyle, as eating better gives you more energy. The nutritional information in the restaurant listings can help you see how you're doing in your day and where you need to make some changes. Table 4 (on page 09) shows Canada's Food Guide recommendations for the daily consumption of different types of foods. To maximize your health, choose whole grains over refined or white grains, lower-fat milk products and lean meats.

It's best to increase your fibre by eating more fruits, vegetables and whole grains. Select lean protein and

TWO IN THREE Canadians have one or more of the major risk factors for heart disease, including:

» obesity
» high blood cholesterol
» high triglycerides
» high blood pressure
» smoking
» type 2 diabetes
» poor nutrition
» inactivity
» stress
» heredity

08 Canadian Diabetes Association. Children and Type 2 Diabetes. http://www.diabetes.ca/diabetes-and-you/youth/type2/
09 Canadian Cancer Encyclopedia. http://info.cancer.ca/cce-ecc/ default.aspx?cceid=5425&se=yes&Lang=E
10 Heart and Stroke Foundation. http://www.heartandstroke.com/site/c.ikIQLcMWJtE/ b.3483991/k.34A8/Statistics.htm

NUTRIENT	WOMEN (aged 24-50)	WOMEN (over 50)	MEN (over 24)
CALORIES	2,000	2,000 or less	2,700
PROTEIN	50 g	50 g or less	63 g
FAT	65 g or less	65 g or less	88 g or less
SATURATED FAT	20 g or less	20 g or less	27 g or less
CARBOHYDRATES	304 g	304 g	410 g
FIBRE	25-35 g	25-35 g	25-35 g
CHOLESTEROL	300 mg or less	300 mg or less	300 mg or less
IRON	18 mg	8 mg	8 mg
SODIUM	1,500 mg	1,500 mg	1,500 mg
CALCIUM	1,000 mg	1,200 mg	1,000 mg

TABLE 3A: Recommended Daily Nutrition Values for Active Lifestyles
Source: Adapted from The Center for Food Safety and Applied Nutrition and Cooking Light Magazine

NUTRIENT	WOMEN (over 24)	MEN (over 24)
CALORIES	1,600	2,160
PROTEIN	40 g	50 g
FAT	52 g or less	70 g or less
SATURATED FAT	16 g or less	22 g or less
CARBOHYDRATES	243 g	328 g
FIBRE	25-35 g	25-35 g
CHOLESTEROL	300 mg or less	300 mg or less
IRON	8 mg	8 mg
SODIUM	1,500 mg	1,500 mg
CALCIUM	1,200 mg	1,000 mg

TABLE 3B: Recommended Daily Nutrition for Sedentary Lifestyles
Source: Adapted from The Center for Food Safety and Applied Nutrition and Cooking Light Magazine

dairy products with lower percentages of fat. Try eating vegetarian a couple of days per week and select fish over beef on a regular basis. Substitute tofu for meat or poultry for a vegetarian option.

Calories

A calorie is a unit of energy that measures how much energy food provides to the body. The body needs calories to function properly. Food labels list calories by the amount in each serving size. Serving sizes differ from one food to the next, so to figure out how many calories you're eating you'll need to do three things:

» Look at the serving size.
» See how many calories there are in one serving.
» Multiply the number of calories by the number of servings you're going to eat.

Fat

Twenty to 35 percent of the energy you consume each day should come from food with less than 10 percent saturated fat.[11]

11   Health Castle. Nutrition 101: Fat. http://www.healthcastle.com/nutrition101_fat.shtml

What is fat for?

» It provides energy during endurance exercise, in between meals and in times of starvation.
» It's an essential component of cell membranes.
» It insulates and acts as a shock absorber for bones and organs.
» Unsaturated fats ("good fats") decrease one's risk of heart disease.
» Omega-3 fatty acids assist in growth, development and brain function.

Where is fat found?

» Unsaturated fats are found in vegetable oils (used in some salad dressings and margarines), avocadoes, flax seeds and other seeds, nuts and fatty fish such as salmon, sardines and mackerel.
» Saturated fats are found in high-fat cuts of beef and pork and full-fat dairy products, including butter and snack foods such as cookies, pastries and donuts.
» Trans-fats are found in some margarines, deep-fried foods and snack foods such as chips, crackers, pastries and donuts.

	CHILDREN			TEENS		ADULTS			
AGE IN YEARS	2-3	4-8	9-13	14-18		19-50		51+	
SEX	Girls & Boys			Females	Males	Females	Males	Females	Males
VEGETABLES & FRUITS	4	5	6	7	8	7-8	8-10	7	7
GRAIN PRODUCTS	3	4	6	6	7	6-7	8	6	7
MILK & ALTERNATIVES	2	2	3-4	3-4	3-4	2	2	3	3
MEAT & ALTERNATIVES	1	1	1-2	2	3	2	3	2	3

TABLE 4: Recommended Number of Food Guide Servings per Day *Source: Canada's Food Guide. http://www.hc-sc .gc.ca/fn-an/food-guide- aliment/index-eng.php*

Saturated fats are derived from animal products such as meat, dairy and eggs. But they are also found in some plant-based sources such as coconut, palm and palm kernel oils. These fats are solid at room temperature. Saturated fats directly raise total and LDL (bad) cholesterol levels. Conventional advice says to avoid them as much as possible, but recently some have questioned this, as certain saturated fats have been found to have at least a neutral effect on cholesterol.

Cholesterol is a fat (lipid) produced by the liver and is crucial for normal body functioning. It exists in the outer layer of every cell in our body and has many functions:

» It builds and maintains cell membranes.
» It is involved in the production of sex hormones (androgens and estrogens).
» It is essential for the production of hormones released by the adrenal glands (cortisol, corticosterone, aldosterone and others).
» It aids in the production of bile.
» It converts sunshine to vitamin D.
» It is important for the metabolism of fat-soluble vitamins, including vitamins A, D, E and K.
» It insulates nerve fibres.

Sodium

Sodium is necessary to regulate blood pressure and fluid volume and helps maintain pH balance. Your muscles and nervous system also need sodium to function properly. However, Canadians eat about 3,400 mg of sodium each day, which is more than *double* the amount we need. The recommended amount for adults is approximately 1,500 mg and for children less than 1,000 mg daily.[12] Our government was working to regulate the amount of salt food manufacturers use, but that agenda has come to a halt with little explanation. Most likely, pressure from food companies and the time and money required to make these changes have stalled the advancement of new salt regulations.[13]

Sodium is an essential nutrient found in salt and many foods. Our bodies need a small amount of sodium to be healthy, but too much can lead to high blood pressure, a major risk factor for stroke, heart disease and kidney disease. Sodium intake has also been linked to an increased risk for osteoporosis, stomach cancer and greater severity of asthma.

12   Health Canada. Sodium in Canada. http://www.hc-sc.gc.ca/ fn-an/nutrition/sodium/index-eng.php
13   *Globe and Mail.* "Sodium Reduction: A Proud Moment That Went Nowhere." January 11, 2012. http://www .theglobeandmail.com/news/opinions/editorials/ sodium-reduction-a-proud-moment-that-went- nowhere/article2299353/

Where the salt comes from in our diet is interesting. Seventy-seven percent is added to packed, processed food and items served in restaurants, 12 percent occurs naturally in foods and 5 percent is added when cooking. Only 6 percent is added during meals. So keeping the salt shaker on the table is not as bad as eating out.[14]

Carbohydrates

Complex carbohydrates include fruits, vegetables, nuts, diary products and whole grains. They supply energy to our bodies. Women with active lifestyles need between 300 and 400 grams of carbohydrates daily; men can have more. But we often get much more than the recommendation because of our affinity for simple carbs, including, sugar, desserts and white grains.

CANADA: A FAST-FOOD NATION

Fast food has been around since the 1950s. On any given day, about 25 percent of Canadians eat a fast-food meal. Many of our calories come from restaurants and packaged or frozen meals, and many are eaten outside the home. No cooking, no thinking, no mess or cleanup.

But we are paying a dear price with our health for this unnecessary convenience. Many of us are addicted to the fat, salt and sugar found in fast food. Once we are hooked, fast food is tough to get away from. It's delicious, inexpensive and convenient. But this quick fix is killing us! How can we learn to select healthier items at restaurants? The answer lies in selecting fast-food meals that are better for you yet still tasty and filling enough to leave you satisfied.

A lot of people start a diet and lose weight, but once they go off their diet they gain it all back. This is because diets work on the basis of deprivation and often eliminate entire food groups such as carbohydrates. Anyone can lose weight, but maintaining that weight loss is the key. Instead of preaching, I say let's meet halfway. Take baby steps before you walk. Letting go of your food addictions will put you on the right path to selecting healthier items.

Choose It and Lose It gives you a popular unhealthy food choice, shows you the calories, fat and saturated fat, carbohydrates and sodium and gives you a better but still tasty choice.

THE FUTURE OF FAST FOOD

Restaurants are becoming concerned with all the "noise" over the connection between food, weight and chronic disease. Many are becoming more proactive—some because they care about their customers and anticipate increased demand for healthier fare and others because they're concerned that changing consumer demand combined with the demand from the health community will ultimately lead to mandatory legislation on healthier options.

The trend towards healthier eating and less-processed food is here to stay. Just look at the increased demand for organic and local food. In 2007, 45 percent of households reported that they often or sometimes bought organic food, and 5 percent bought organic food all the time.[15] I believe that in the future more restaurants will offer healthier fats and more fruits and vegetables at affordable prices.

We all know that eating food prepared from scratch in our own kitchens is the best way to go. But the reality today is that this is nearly impossible for many people. *Choose It and Lose It,* while not endorsing a daily diet of fast food, demonstrates that you can make better choices at restaurants and ultimately lose weight without feeling deprived. Small daily changes can lead to a lifetime of better health.

---

14   Health Canada. Sodium in Canada. http://www.hc-sc.gc.ca /fn-an/nutrition/sodium/index-eng.php

15   Agriculture and Agri-Food Canada. http://www.statcan.gc.ca /pub/16-201-x/2009000/part-partie1-eng.htm

MYTHS ABOUT EATING IN RESTAURANTS

CHICKEN AND FISH DISHES ARE ALWAYS GOOD CHOICES FOR DIETERS.

Chicken and fish are lower in calories, overall fat and saturated fat than red meat, but fried or battered dishes will always have excess calories and often come with additional butter, cream or cheese sauces.

RED MEAT DISHES ARE NOT GOOD CHOICES FOR HEALTH-CONSCIOUS DINERS.

Most red meat dishes contain more fat than chicken or fish, but if you select lean cuts with visible fat trimmed away, you can enjoy 3 to 4 ounces (90 to 125 grams) with your meals—even on a *daily* basis. The problem is that most restaurant portions are larger and fattier than necessary. You can always share an entrée or take half home. Start your meal with a salad (with dressing on the side) or a soup that's not cream based. Either will fill you up enough that a smaller portion of beef will suffice.

VEGETARIAN DISHES ARE ALWAYS HEALTHY.

We should all be consuming more vegetables and fruits, but vegetarianism is not always the answer. Many meatless dishes contain loads of fat, cheese, oil or nuts, and they can be very high in calories, overall fat and even saturated fat.

IT'S IMPOSSIBLE TO "EAT HEALTHY" AT FAST-FOOD RESTAURANTS.

Most fast-food restaurants today offer healthy options. Ask the server for those items or ask for substitutions.

GUIDELINES FOR EATING OUT

If you allow yourself to eat out regularly, you have to know how to count calories, fat, sugar and sodium for your day and how restaurant offerings fit into your specific equation. Here are some guidelines:

» Feel full on fewer calories, but more food.
» Have 3 ounces (85 grams) of lean protein, such as skinless chicken, beef, fish or tofu, at each meal.
» Remove the skin from chicken and trim beef fat.
» Say no to extra cheese.
» Avoid deep-fried foods and heavily marbled meats. Go for grilled and ask how it's prepared.
» Limit the amount of animal fat you eat.
» Try a non-cream-based soup or salad (dressing on the side) to begin your meal. This prevents overeating.
» Watch out for the "freebies" given out at restaurants, such as bread and butter, nuts, nachos, dips or olives.
» Watch your intake of simple carbohydrates (breads, pastas and sugars).
» Ask for sauces and dressings on the side.

» Avoid combos or value meals.
» Load your burgers or sandwiches with veggies and non-fat condiments such as mustard, ketchup and relish. Avoid mayonnaise and "special" or "secret" sauces.
» Avoid drinking your calories.
» Remember that children's or kids' meals are usually unhealthy. They often have excess cheese and come with complimentary sugary beverages or refills.
» Don't deprive yourself in restaurants. Alter your meal to make it healthier.
» Ask the server how the meal is prepared.

LEARN THE LINGO

→

Restaurant and fast-food options have a vocabulary of their own. Decoding these words will allow you to make healthier choices.

WORST DESCRIPTORS

» **Complimentary** chips, breads, refills or desserts are low-cost foods the restaurant gives away to make you think you're getting great value.
» **Creamy** always means butter or cream has been added.
» **Crispy** or **crunchy** usually means deep-fried and breaded. Think of food described like this as bathed in oil!
» **Italian cold cuts** are cured fatty meats with excess sodium. These include ham, salami, pepperoni, prosciutto and mortadella.
» **Pan-fried** or **sautéed** usually means that excess oil has been used.
» **Prime** meat is heavily marbled and contains up to 50 percent more calories and fat than leaner cuts.

» **Secret** or **special sauce** is either mayonnaise or oil based.
» **Stuffed pizza crusts** or **deep-dish crusts** have loads of unnecessary bread or simple carbs.
» **Supersize** meals (watch the movie *Supersize Me!*) can have 50 percent more calories and fat than the next size down.
» **Tempura** is just a Japanese word for deep-fried and battered.
» **Wraps** can have 300 calories in the tortilla alone, which is more than two slices of bread. The condiments added to any wrap, such as extra cheese, dressing, mayonnaise or sour cream, can add up to 50 percent more calories.

BEST DESCRIPTORS

» **Create your own** meals can be great alternatives if you know what to select.
» Anything **grilled, poached, roasted, steamed** or **baked** tends to use less fat.

» **Vinaigrette dressing** is still packed with a 3:1 ratio of oil to vinegar, but it usually has fewer calories than mayonnaise-, cheese- or oil-based dressings such as caesar, blue cheese or thousand island.

WHAT TO WATCH OUT FOR IN DIFFERENT

ITALIAN

What to avoid
› deli meats and extra cheese on your pizza
› cream- and cheese-based pasta sauces such as alfredo or rosé
› cream-based soups
› garlic bread
› dressed caesar salads
› antipasto salads with smoked meats, olives and oil-bathed veggies
› fried calamari
› pastas stuffed with fatty meats and topped with heavy or creamy sauces such as lasagna, tortellini, ravioli, manicotti and cannelloni
› chicken or veal parmesan, usually deep-fried and breaded
› risotto, always loaded with butter, excess oil and cheese
› tiramisu, made with mascarpone cheese, which contains **45 percent** milk fat! Forgetaboutit!

What to order
› minestrone or bean soups
› thin-crust pizza
› salads with dressing on the side
› bread with olive oil and balsamic vinegar
› mussels marinara
› grilled calamari
› steamed clams or mussels
› pastas with a tomato, pesto or stock-based sauce
› meat or fish in tomato, wine or stock-based sauce
› thin-crust pizza with vegetables and minimal cheese
› fruit sorbet or Italian ice

CHINESE

What to avoid
› egg rolls
› fried rice—often made with shortening or lard
› sweet and sour dishes
› spareribs—the fattiest food in Chinese cuisine
› regular soy sauce, which is high in sodium

What to order
› hot and sour soup
› Chinese vegetable or steamed pork wonton soup
› stir-fried dishes made with minimal oil
› stir-fried chicken, seafood, vegetable and tofu dishes
› steamed fish or chicken
› steamed white rice with low-sodium soy sauce and vegetables
› low-sodium soy sauce

INDIAN

What to avoid
› coconut milk–based soups or dishes
› samosas
› curries made with coconut milk

What to order
› bean or lentil soups, which are usually stock or tomato based
› tandoori chicken, beef or fish dishes baked in a yogurt sauce
› shish kebabs—meat, fish and vegetables baked or grilled with spices and a marinade
› rice pilaf or steamed rice
› fruit or vegetable chutneys

YPES OF RESTAURANTS

JAPANESE

What to avoid
› fish or vegetable tempura
› fried tofu
› excess full-sodium soy sauce
› sushi made with mayonnaise

What to order
› miso soup—a fish-based soup with soybean paste, tofu and seaweed
› sushi and sashimi—sashimi is raw fish minus the sushi rice
› yakitori—shish kebabs made with meat, chicken or fish
› shabu-shabu—sliced meat with noodles and vegetables
› teriyaki dishes with meat, seafood or tofu
› steamed rice
› tofu that has not been fried

FRENCH

What to avoid
› traditional sauces such as hollandaise, béchamel and Bearnaise
› quiche Lorraine
› French onion soup with heavy cheese topping
› cream-based soups
› cheese fondues
› duck, goose and pâtés
› gratin dishes

What to order
› consommés
› sauces made with wine
› poached or steamed fish

NORTH AMERICAN

What to avoid
› nachos with cheese sauce
› hot dogs
› fried chicken
› french fries
› loaded hamburgers
› pizza with deli meats, extra cheese and thick or filled crusts
› ice cream and milk shakes

What to order
› grilled or roasted chicken (remove skin)
› thin-crust pizza
› grilled chicken or veggie burgers
› salads with plain proteins and dressing on the side
› baked potatoes with grated cheese, vegetables and light sour cream
› kebabs and rice
› pastas with tomato sauce
› frozen yogurt and low-fat ice cream

STEAK HOUSE

What to avoid
› marbled fatty steaks such as prime rib and rib-eye
› fried potatoes or potato gratin

What to order
› top sirloin, New York strip or filet mignon
› baked or steamed potatoes

DELICATESSEN

What to avoid

› deli meats, such as corned beef, pastrami
  and salami, which have excess sodium and
  fat and contain nitrites and nitrates (cancer-
  causing agents)
› latkes or potato pancakes, which are
  cooked with excess oil
› potato salad or coleslaw made with large
  amounts of mayonnaise or oil
› hot dogs
› chicken soup with matzo balls, which
  are made with chicken fat

What to order

› roasted meats such as turkey, roast beef
  or chicken
› chicken soup with noodles or rice

MEXICAN

What to avoid

› tortilla chips and taco shells
› refried beans
› quesadillas, burritos and enchiladas,
  if filled with fatty meat, excess cheese
  and sour cream
› excess guacamole
› taco salad in a fried tortilla shell

What to order

› baked tortilla chips served with salsa
  and low-fat sour cream
› fajitas, soft tacos or burritos made with
  chicken, beef or seafood and lots of vegetables,
  with added salsa, low-fat sour cream and a
  small amount of cheese
› gazpacho—a cold tomato-based vegetable soup
› vegetable-based burritos and enchiladas
  with small amounts of cheese
› salads with the dressing on the side

RESTAURANT LISTINGS

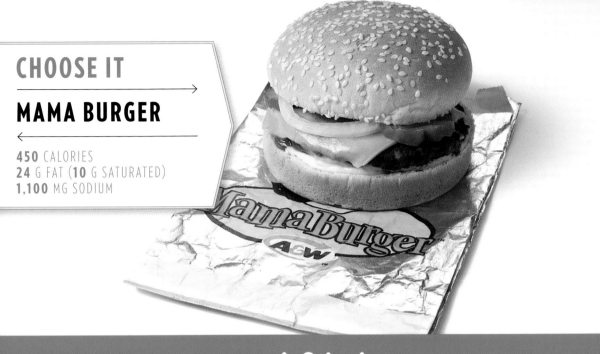

CHOOSE IT

→

MAMA BURGER

←

450 CALORIES
24 G FAT (**10** G SATURATED)
1,100 MG SODIUM

A&W

In 1919, California entrepreneur Roy Allen created the original creamy root beer. In 1922, Allen and his business partner, Frank Wright, opened A&W, which they named after themselves. Thus began the chain that is now worldwide. The first drive-in A&W restaurant in Canada opened in 1956. Today there are over 700 locations throughout the country. The menu primarily consists of burgers, fries and breakfast items. The A&W website features an excellent nutritional calculator and lists the ingredients used in all its items.

Why choose it? The Mama Burger has the fewest calories and lowest fat content out of all A&W's Burger Family sandwiches, mainly because of the absence of bacon and the inclusion of the teen sauce, which lists water rather than oil as its first ingredient.

ALSO CHOOSE

BREAKFAST:
Bacon 'n' Egger
› **430** calories
› **27** g fat
 (**8** g saturated)
› **900** mg sodium

SIDES:
Onion Rings
› **470** calories
› **27** g fat
 (**2** g saturated)
› **780** mg sodium

CHICKEN:
Grilled Chicken Deluxe
› **320** calories
› **9** g fat
 (**1.5** g saturated)
› **1,040** mg sodium

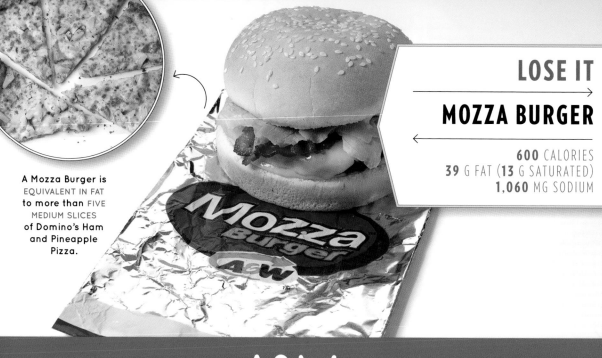

A Mozza Burger is EQUIVALENT IN FAT to more than FIVE MEDIUM SLICES of Domino's Ham and Pineapple Pizza.

MOZZA BURGER

600 CALORIES
39 G FAT (**13** G SATURATED)
1,060 MG SODIUM

A&W

Why lose it? This 100 percent beef patty has bacon and Mozza sauce, which is made primarily with oil and packs on extra calories and fat. This burger alone adds up to one-third of the daily recommended calorie intake and more than half the daily recommended fat intake for women.

ALSO LOSE

BREAKFAST:
Homestyle Ham 'n' Egger
› **595** calories
› **40** g fat
  (**11** g saturated)
› **1,140** mg sodium

SIDES:
Poutine
› **740** calories
› **40** g fat
  (**12** g saturated)
› **1,880** mg sodium

CHICKEN:
Chubby Chicken
› **480** calories
› **26** g fat
  (**3** g saturated)
› **1,230** mg sodium

HOME COOKING

Most restaurants use a fattier grade of ground beef for their burgers, which customers seem to prefer. There are around 300 calories, 23 g of fat and 9 g of saturated fat in 4 oz (113 g) of regular ground beef. Now add bacon, cheese and heavy sauces, and you'll understand why a restaurant burger is loaded with calories and fat. At home, I use 4 oz (113 g) of lean ground beef, which has only 200 calories, 7 g of fat and 3 g of saturated fat, and then load the burger up with sliced tomatoes, lettuce and non-fat condiments. A nutritional bargain!

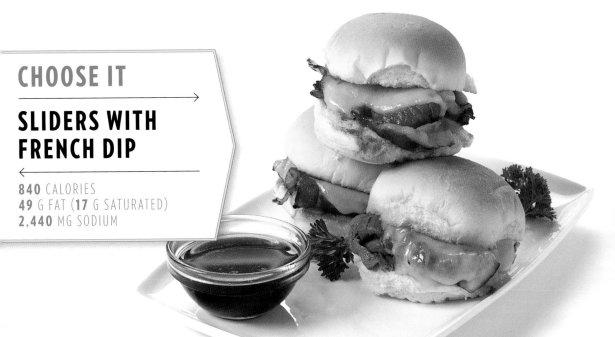

CHOOSE IT

SLIDERS WITH FRENCH DIP

840 CALORIES
49 G FAT (**17** G SATURATED)
2,440 MG SODIUM

APPLEBEE'S

With over 2,000 restaurants internationally, Applebee's is the largest casual dining restaurant chain in the world and has locations across Canada. The menu caters to a wide variety of customers, with creative appetizers, salads, ribs, chicken, burgers, sandwiches and an "under 550 calories" section, featuring dishes such as Asiago Peppercorn Steak, Grilled Dijon Chicken & Portobello and Teriyaki Shrimp Pasta. Applebee's Canada currently does not have nutritional information available on its website, so the analysis here was taken from the U.S. site.

Why choose it? These roast beef and cheese sliders (served with jus) have less fat and sodium and fewer calories than the clubhouse—due to the ground beef versus the smoked meat as well as the mayo and BBQ sauce on the Classic Clubhouse Grill. Enjoy a side salad or soup to make a complete meal.

ALSO CHOOSE

APPETIZER:
Classic Wings, Southern BBQ
› **660** calories
› **35** g fat
   (**9** g saturated)
› **1,060** mg sodium

SALAD:
Grilled Chicken Caesar
(regular)
› **820** calories
› **57** g fat
   (**11** g saturated)
› **1,740** mg sodium

CHICKEN:
Grilled Dijon Chicken & Portobello
› **470** calories
› **16** g fat
   (**7** g saturated)
› **1,820** mg sodium

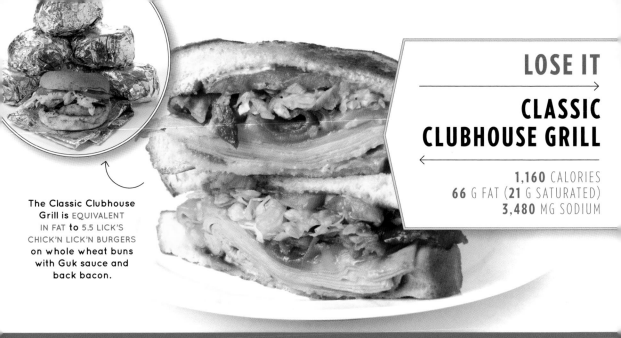

CLASSIC CLUBHOUSE GRILL

1,160 CALORIES
66 G FAT (**21** G SATURATED)
3,480 MG SODIUM

The Classic Clubhouse Grill is EQUIVALENT IN FAT to 5.5 LICK'S CHICK'N LICK'N BURGERS on whole wheat buns with Guk sauce and back bacon.

APPLEBEE'S

Why lose it? You don't need so many varieties of fatty proteins in one sandwich. Ham, two cheeses and smoked bacon give you excess calories, fat and sodium. With a day's worth of fat and two day's worth of sodium, you should definitely lose this.

HEALTH WARNING

Both nitrates and nitrites are used extensively to cure, and enhance the colour and extend the shelf life of processed meats. Processed meats, including hot dogs, salami, sausages and other deli meats, have been linked to colon, stomach and bladder cancer. Minimize your daily consumption of these types of meats.

ALSO LOSE

APPETIZER:
Spinach & Artichoke Dip
› **1,560** calories
› **100** g fat
  (**27** g saturated)
› **2,630** mg sodium

SALAD:
Oriental Chicken Salad
(regular)
› **1,380** calories
› **99** g fat
  (**15** g saturated)
› **1,430** mg sodium

CHICKEN:
Fiesta Lime Chicken
› **1,200** calories
› **66** g fat
  (**16** g saturated)
› **3,030** mg sodium

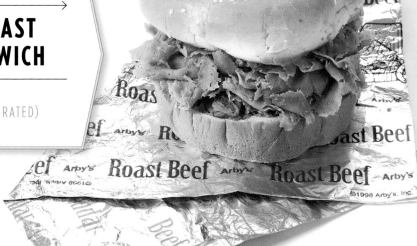

CHOOSE IT

CLASSIC ROAST BEEF SANDWICH

340 CALORIES
13 G FAT (**4.5** G SATURATED)
930 MG SODIUM

ARBY'S

Arby's first opened in 1964 in Boardman, Ohio, and now has over 3,600 restaurants in the United States, Canada, Turkey, Qatar and the United Arab Emirates. Arby's got its name from the initials R.B., which stands for the Raffel brothers, and not, as many believe, for roast beef. The menu offers a wide variety of American-style meals. I have to admire that Arby's, in 1994, was the first chain restaurant to ban smoking! Plus, the website provides nutritional information, ingredients, gluten-free menu items and a list of allergens.

Why choose it? Lean sliced roast beef is a great calorie and fat saver. Arby's Sauce is tomato based rather than mayonnaise based.

ALSO CHOOSE

SANDWICH:
Philly Beef & Swiss
› **410** calories
› **19** g fat
  (**8** g saturated)
› **1,150** mg sodium

SIDEKICKERS:
Turkey Club Salad
(including Italian dressing)
› **350** calories
› **23** g fat
  (**8.5** g saturated)
› **1,470** mg sodium

CHILDREN'S MEAL:
Junior Roast Beef Combo
(including small-size homestyle fries)
› **420** calories
› **16** g fat
  (**4** g saturated)
› **990** mg sodium

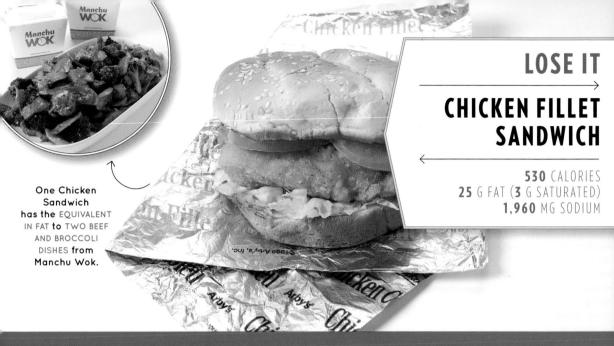

One Chicken Sandwich has the EQUIVALENT IN FAT to TWO BEEF AND BROCCOLI DISHES from Manchu Wok.

LOSE IT

→

CHICKEN FILLET SANDWICH

←

530 CALORIES
25 G FAT (**3** G SATURATED)
1,960 MG SODIUM

ARBY'S

Why lose it? The name of the sandwich doesn't indicate that the chicken is deep-fried, which raises the calories and doubles the fat. The addition of mayonnaise is another reason to pass on this sandwich. As if that weren't enough, it contains over a day's sodium.

ALSO LOSE

SANDWICH:
Ultimate BLT Sandwich
› **670** calories
› **42** g fat (**8** g saturated)
› **1,360** mg sodium

SIDEKICKERS:
Chopped Farmhouse Crispy Chicken Salad
(including French dressing)
› **640** calories
› **43** g fat (**12** g saturated)
› **1,500** mg sodium

CHILDREN'S MEAL:
Kid's Chicken Tender Combo
(including small-size curly fries)
› **520** calories
› **28** g fat (**4** g saturated)
› **1,310** mg sodium

NUTRITION

Much of the roast beef in restaurants or in the deli department of your supermarket is high in sodium because it's been processed. Meat that has been traditionally roasted, then sliced, is a much better choice. Luckily, many of the better-quality supermarkets offer fresh-roasted meats. Three ounces (85 g) of deli-style roast beef contain approximately 1,200 mg of sodium; there's only 56 mg of sodium in oven-roasted beef without the additives. Making roast beef at home keeps the sodium to a minimum—a good way to prevent high blood pressure.

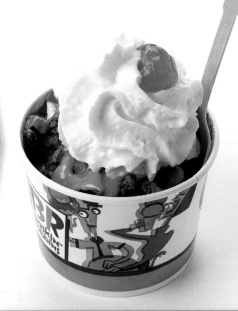

CHOOSE IT

→

31 Below
REESE'S PEANUT BUTTER CUPS
(small 12 oz/340 g)

640 CALORIES
29 G FAT (**15** G SATURATED)
84 G CARBOHYDRATES
78 G SUGAR

BASKIN ROBBINS

Baskin Robbins was started over 75 years ago by brothers-in-law Burt Baskin and Irv Robbins, who wanted to create a neighbourhood ice cream shop. With over 5,600 stores in 40 countries, the company continues to grow. BR is famous for its 31 flavours—one for every day of the month—as well as its pink tasting spoons. BR offers seasonal flavours, soft ice cream with mix-ins, ice cream cakes, sundaes and beverages. For the calorie conscious, they offer low-fat yogurt, no-sugar sorbets, sherbets and light ice cream flavours. Nutritional information is from the U.S. website.

Why choose it? The lower-calorie soft ice cream uses non-fat milk and a small amount of cream instead of Baskin Robbins's regular hard ice cream, which is cream and high-fat milk based. So go ahead and enjoy the peanut butter sauce and chunks—but only as an occasional treat.

ALSO CHOOSE

ICE CREAM VS. SMOOTHIES:	SHAKES:	CONES:
Jamoca Ice Cream Scoop (medium)	**Strawberry Shake** (medium, including Very Berry Strawberry ice cream)	**Cake Cone** (7 g)
› **260** calories	› **780** calories	› **25** calories
› **15** g fat (7 g saturated)	› **31** g fat (20 g saturated)	› **0** g fat
› **29** g carbohydrates	› **109** g carbohydrates	› **5** g carbohydrates
› **23** g sugar	› **106** g sugar	› **0** g sugar

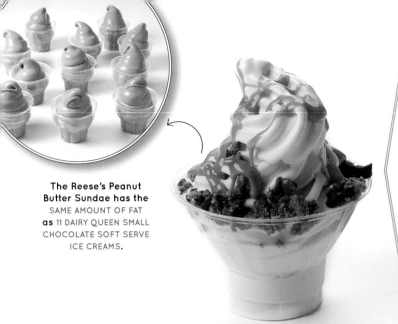

The Reese's Peanut Butter Sundae has the SAME AMOUNT OF FAT as 11 DAIRY QUEEN SMALL CHOCOLATE SOFT SERVE ICE CREAMS.

LOSE IT

Sundae

REESE'S PEANUT BUTTER CUPS
(12 oz/340 g)

1,220 CALORIES
80 G FAT (**32** G SATURATED)
109 G CARBOHYDRATES
92 G SUGAR

BASKIN ROBBINS

Why lose it? At Baskin Robbins, a triple layer of anything spells trouble. This sundae equals close to three-quarters of a day's calories, over a day's fat, 1.5 days' saturated fat and two days' sugar. Clogged arteries, here we come!

TRIVIA

Japan has over 850 Baskin Robbins locations, the highest number outside of the United States. After Japan comes Korea, the Middle East and Latin America. The top-selling flavours are Vanilla (representing 25 percent of selected flavours), Chocolate, Mint Chocolate Chip, Pralines 'n' Cream and Chocolate Chip.

ALSO LOSE

ICE CREAM VS. SMOOTHIES:
Mango Banana Smoothie
(medium)
› **630** calories
› **2** g fat
  (**0** g saturated)
› **150** g carbohydrates
› **134** g sugar

SHAKES:
Chocolate Chip Cookie Dough Shake
(medium)
› **980** calories
› **42** g fat
  (**27** g saturated)
› **131** g carbohydrates
› **114** g sugar

CONES:
Waffle Cone
(38 g)
› **160** calories
› **4** g fat
  (**1** g saturated)
› **28** g carbohydrates
› **13** g sugar

CHOOSE IT

DELUXE HAMBURGER
(8 oz/226 g)

860 CALORIES
53 G FAT (**13** G SATURATED)
740 MG SODIUM

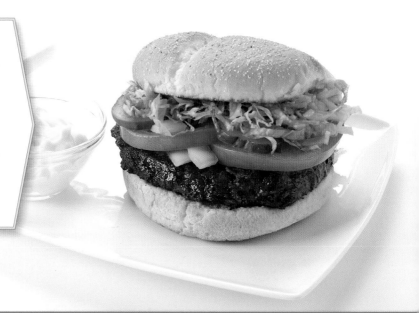

BATON ROUGE

Since opening in 1992, Baton Rouge, with its elegant atmosphere, is perfect for special celebrations, cocktails with friends or an intimate evening for two. It offers AAA steaks, barbecue back ribs, seafood, salads, appetizers and decadent desserts. Baton Rouge's website features a link to nutritional information on its homepage. This information is organized by meal type.

Why choose it? You get two more ounces of meat than with the Louisiana Chicken Sandwich and a garnish of mayo. The burger has just over half the sodium of the chicken sandwich.

ALSO CHOOSE

GRILL:
New York Strip Loin
(10 oz/283 g)
› **580** calories
› **26** g fat
   (**10** g saturated)
› **160** mg sodium

PORK:
Pork Chops
(14 oz/397 g)
› **830** calories
› **44** g fat
   (**14** g saturated)
› **220** mg sodium

ENTRÉE SALADS:
Seared Ahi Tuna Salad
(including lime dressing)
› **490** calories
› **17** g fat
   (**6** g saturated)
› **500** mg sodium

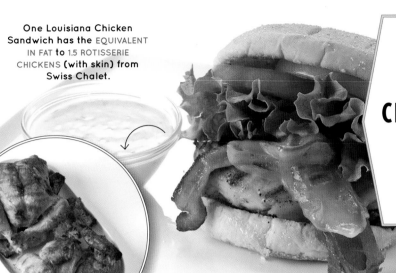

One Louisiana Chicken Sandwich has the EQUIVALENT IN FAT to 1.5 ROTISSERIE CHICKENS (with skin) from Swiss Chalet.

LOUISIANA CHICKEN SANDWICH
(6 oz/170 g)

1,290 CALORIES
95 G FAT (**17** G SATURATED)
1,340 MG SODIUM

BATON ROUGE

Why lose it? Even though the chicken is grilled, the addition of smoked bacon, Monterey Jack cheese and creamy Dijonnaise sauce ramps up the calories and fat so that you're getting ¾ of a day's calories, a day's sodium and 1½ days' of fat. Not much left for the rest of your day!

ALSO LOSE

GRILL:
Louisiana BBQ Chicken
(10 oz/283 g, including barbecue sauce)
› **970** calories
› **71** g fat
   (**7** g saturated)
› **1,200** mg sodium

PORK:
BBQ Pork Back Ribs
(10 oz/283 g, including barbecue sauce)
› **1,160** calories
› **77** g fat
   (**30** g saturated)
› **820** mg sodium

ENTRÉE SALADS:
Louisiana Chicken Salad
(including dressing, peanut sauce, noodles)
› **900** calories
› **48** g fat
   (**9** g saturated)
› **1,240** mg sodium

EXERCISE

If you're going to indulge in the Louisiana Chicken Sandwich, consider walking to the restaurant and back, and then walk some more! You'll need to walk at a moderate speed for five hours to burn off the 1,290 calories and 95 g of fat!

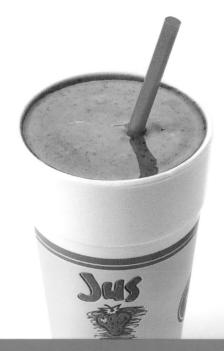

BERRY CREAM SENSATION

325 CALORIES
3 G FAT
5 G PROTEIN

BOOSTER JUICE

Booster Juice is Canada's largest chain of fresh juice and smoothie bars, with over 200 stores worldwide. The idea for Canada's premier juice bar chain was born during a 1999 camping trip future founder Jon Amack and Dale Wishewan took. The menu is known for its wide range of smoothies. Most smoothies are made with a combination of fresh fruit, yogurt, frozen vanilla yogurt or sorbets. All beverages listed here are 24 oz (680 g). You won't find the nutritional information online; you'll have to go to the counter in the restaurant and ask to look at a binder. There are no information pamphlets.

Why choose it? You're getting a wide variety of fruit in this smoothie, adding to the nutrients without packing on extra fat, calories or sugar. It has only 5 g of protein, but you don't need a beverage to supply your daily protein if it means adding fat and calories to the package.

ALSO CHOOSE

SMOOTHIES:
Banana Beach
› **225** calories
› **1** g fat
› **4** g protein

HIGH-PROTEIN
SUPERFOOD:
Pomegranate Punch
› **370** calories
› **4** g fat
› **20** g protein

TROPICAL:
Bahama Freeze
› **305** calories
› **0** g fat
› **3** g protein

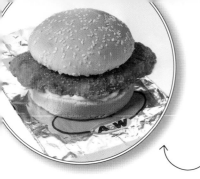

One Funky Monkey is
EQUIVALENT IN CALORIES to ONE
CHUBBY CHICKEN SANDWICH
from A&W.

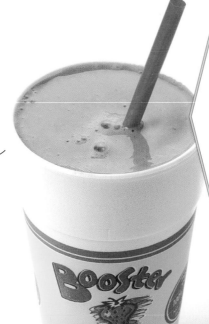

FUNKY MONKEY

585 CALORIES
9 G FAT
20 G PROTEIN

BOOSTER JUICE

Why lose it? The name Funky Monkey doesn't tell you much, but its combination of chocolate soy milk and vanilla frozen yogurt adds calories, fat and refined sugar to this smoothie. It's an excellent source of protein, but you could get the same in 3 oz (85 g) of chicken breast, without all the fat and calories.

ALSO LOSE

SMOOTHIES:
Cranberry Cycle
› **505** calories
› **5** g fat
› **8** g protein

HIGH-PROTEIN
SUPERFOOD:
High Impact Acai
› **580** calories
› **10** g fat
› **25** g protein

TROPICAL:
Pineapple Freeze
› **405** calories
› **5** g fat
› **8** g protein

HOME COOKING

Make a great-tasting smoothie at home with fewer calories and less fat. Combine 1 cup (250 mL) of chocolate milk (one percent milk fat), 1 cup (250 mL) low-fat vanilla yogurt, 1 medium banana, 2 Tbsp (30 mL) honey and 1 Tbsp (15 mL) cocoa powder in a blender. In a one-cup serving (250 mL), you'll get 281 calories, 2.4 g of fat and 10 g of protein. A great breakfast idea!

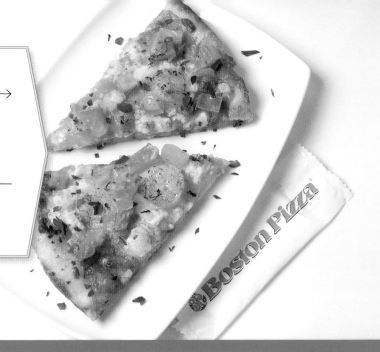

CHOOSE IT

BBQ CHICKEN PIZZA
(2 slices)

380 CALORIES
12 G FAT (**6** G SATURATED)
640 MG SODIUM

BOSTON PIZZA

Canadian chain Boston Pizza opened in Edmonton in 1964 and now has over 325 locations from coast to coast. It has also expanded into the United States and Mexico. With over 100 menu items, BP is much more than a pizzeria. It also offers wings, pastas, sandwiches, salads, entrées and desserts. Recently, BP added "Delicious Alternatives"—healthy items—to its menu. The website organizes nutritional information by type of meal.

Why choose it? Even though chicken is higher in calories and fat than shrimp, the barbecue and tomato sauce on the crust are not dense in calories or fat. Using only two cheeses rather than three also cuts down the fat, calories and sodium.

ALSO CHOOSE

CHICKEN:
Chipotle Chicken Caesar Wrap
› **590** calories
› **27** g fat
  (**5** g saturated)
› **870** mg sodium

PIZZA:
Hawaiian
(individual size,
8 inches/20 cm)
› **780** calories
› **21** g fat
  (**10** g saturated)
› **2,290** mg sodium

SANDWICH:
New York Strip Sandwich
› **420** calories
› **17** g fat
  (**7** g saturated)
› **710** mg sodium

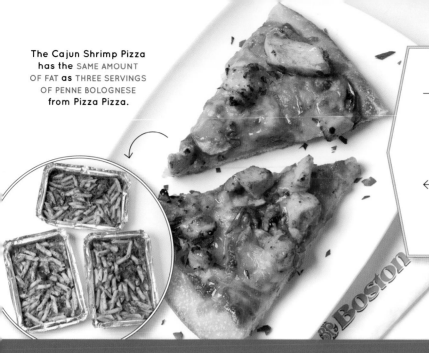

The Cajun Shrimp Pizza **has the** SAME AMOUNT OF FAT **as** THREE SERVINGS OF PENNE BOLOGNESE from Pizza Pizza.

CAJUN SHRIMP PIZZA
(2 slices)

580 CALORIES
30 G FAT (**10** G SATURATED)
1,180 MG SODIUM

BOSTON PIZZA

Why lose it? The creamy garlic and sundried tomato sauce on the crust indicates either an oil- or mayonnaise-based sauce, which boosts the calories and fat. Sundried tomatoes are packed with sodium!

ALSO LOSE

CHICKEN:
Oven-Roasted Chicken Quesadilla
› **940** calories
› **47** g fat
   (**14** g saturated)
› **1,330** mg sodium

PIZZA:
The Great White North
(individual size, 8 inches/20 cm)
› **970** calories
› **39** g fat
   (**22** g saturated)
› **2,740** mg sodium

SANDWICH:
Chicken Ciabatta Sandwich
› **760** calories
› **42** g fat
   (**7** g saturated)
› **1,270** mg sodium

HEALTH WARNING

Watch out for sundried tomatoes! One cup (250 mL) of sundried tomatoes not packed in oil has 140 calories and 1.5 g of fat; 1 cup (250 mL) of sundried tomatoes soaked in olive oil (which is the kind most restaurants use) contains 234 calories and 15 g of fat. One cup contains 1,100 mg of sodium, which is three-quarters of your recommended daily intake.

CHOOSE IT

DOUBLE STACKER

510 CALORIES
32 G FAT (**12** G SATURATED)
750 MG SODIUM

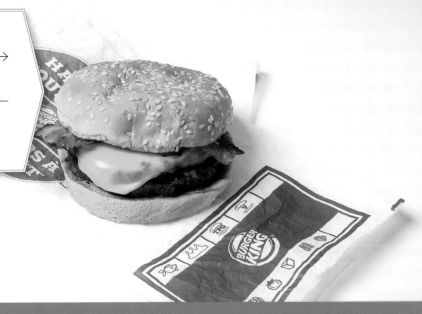

BURGER KING

The Burger King franchise was started in 1954 with its famous flame-broiled beef burger. The King caricature was introduced in 1955 and the Whopper in 1957. Fifty years later, there are over 12,200 outlets in 73 countries around the world. The motto is still "Have it your way," meaning that every burger can be your own creation. The menu now offers a variety of Whoppers, chicken sandwiches, poutine and fries, breakfasts and value meals. The nutritional information is clearly presented online.

Why choose it? Who would have thought that two beef patties, cheese and bacon would have fewer calories and less fat and sodium than the Original Chicken Sandwich? The fact that the Double Stacker isn't deep-fried and breaded makes it the healthier option.

ALSO CHOOSE

SNACKS:
Onion Rings
(medium)
› **320** calories
› **17** g fat
  (**3** g saturated)
› **620** mg sodium

DRINKS:
Chocolate Milk
(250 g)
› **170** calories
› **3** g fat
› **28** g sugar

BREAKFAST:
English Muffin
(including egg, cheese, bacon)
› **340** calories
› **14** g fat
› **810** mg sodium

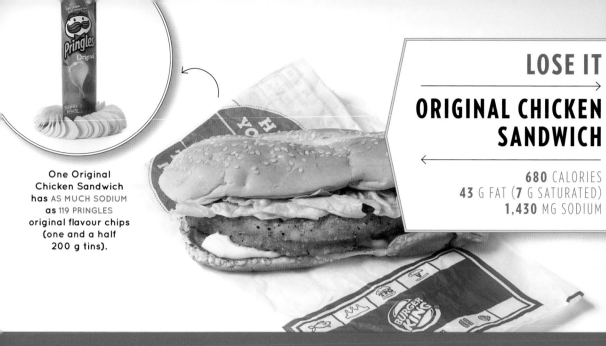

One Original
Chicken Sandwich
has AS MUCH SODIUM
as 119 PRINGLES
original flavour chips
(one and a half
200 g tins).

LOSE IT →

ORIGINAL CHICKEN SANDWICH

680 CALORIES
43 G FAT (**7** G SATURATED)
1,430 MG SODIUM

BURGER KING

Why lose it? The name doesn't tell you it's deep-fried, which always equals higher calories and fat. The day's worth of sodium comes primarily from the chicken breading. Now add a whopping dollop of mayo, and you have almost half of your day's calories and almost your entire daily fat intake in one meal.

ALSO LOSE

SNACKS:
Poutine
> **740** calories
> **41** g fat
  (**15** g saturated)
> **2,500** mg sodium

DRINKS:
Chocolate Shake
(454 g)
> **440** calories
> **7** g fat
> **71** g sugar

BREAKFAST:
English Muffin
(including egg,
cheese, sausage)
> **460** calories
> **26** g fat
> **1,020** mg sodium

HOME COOKING

The best way to have a chicken breast sandwich at home is either to grill the breast, or dip it in an egg and milk wash, then coat it in seasoned bread crumbs or panko crumbs and bake it in a 350°F (175°C) oven until just cooked. A 3 oz (90 g) deep-fried chicken breast has 260 calories and 13 g of fat; a grilled, skinless chicken breast has only 148 calories and 3.5 g of fat.

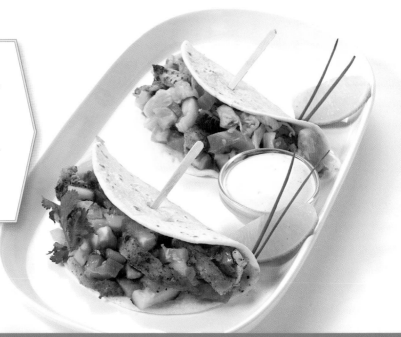

CHOOSE IT →

CHICKEN TACOS
(including dressing)
←

560 CALORIES
33 G FAT (**4** G SATURATED)
900 MG SODIUM

CASEY'S BAR AND GRILL

Casey's Bar and Grill first opened in Sudbury, Ontario, in 1980. Today there are 31 locations in Ontario and Quebec franchised by Prime Restaurants of Canada which also owns Pat and Mario's, East Side Mario's, Prime Pubs and The Bier Markt. There is a wide selection of classic starters, salads, steaks and ribs, burgers and sandwiches, desserts and kids' items, as well as a fairly extensive gluten-free menu and many Health Check items, which are at the top of the nutritional chart. The nutritionals and allergen chart are online and easy to read.

Why choose it? With its lean protein chicken and vegetables, this item is both delicious and filling. The mango salsa and ranch dressing give this taco its flavour.

→

ALSO CHOOSE

PASTA:
Short Rib Rigatoni
(not including garlic bread)
› **740** calories
› **21** g fat
  (**8** g saturated)
› **1,810** mg sodium

SANDWICH:
Steak Sandwich*
› **670** calories
› **36** g fat
  (**12** g saturated)
› **590** mg sodium

DESSERT:
Pecan Pie
(including French vanilla ice cream)
› **830** calories
› **53** g fat
  (**23** g saturated)
› **54** g sugar
› **630** mg sodium

Ontario only

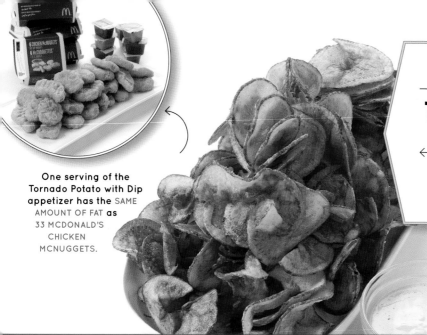

One serving of the Tornado Potato with Dip appetizer has the SAME AMOUNT OF FAT as 33 MCDONALD'S CHICKEN MCNUGGETS.

LOSE IT

TORNADO POTATO
(including dip)

1,330 CALORIES
114 G FAT (**15** G SATURATED)
850 MG SODIUM

CASEY'S BAR AND GRILL

Why lose it? Just another version of french fries but with a Cajun dip, which alone has enough calories and fat to bury this potato starter. With few nutrients to satisfy your hunger and over three-quarters of a day's worth of calories and two days' worth of fat, the Tornado Potato is best shared with at least four of your friends!

WEIGHT LOSS

If you ate at Casey's once a week for a year and chose the Chicken Tacos instead of the Tornado Potato with Dip, you would lose 12 lb (5 kg) without doing anything else. You would also lower your cholesterol and your chance of developing heart disease and type 2 diabetes. Well worth the switch!

ALSO LOSE

PASTA:
Nine Vegetable Linguine
(not including garlic bread)
› **1,180** calories
› **80** g fat
   (**15** g saturated)
› **1,260** mg sodium

SANDWICH:
Clubhouse Sandwich
› **1,040** calories
› **63** g fat
   (**22** g saturated)
› **2,380** mg sodium

DESSERT:
Chocolate Cake*
(including chocolate icing)
› **1,670** calories
› **78** g fat
   (**25** g saturated)
› **162** g sugar
› **1,440** mg sodium

*Ontario only

CHOOSE IT

→

CARIBBEAN SALAD
(including grilled chicken)

←

610 CALORIES
25 G FAT (**4** G SATURATED)
810 MG SODIUM

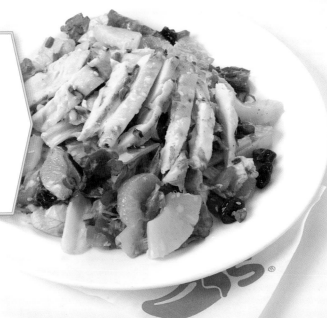

CHILI'S

Chili's opened in 1975 in Dallas as a fun burger joint. Today it is an international chain with more than 1,400 restaurants offering a variety of Tex-Mex-inspired American food. Although most of the menu consists of high-fat indulgences, Chili's also offers healthier items such as the "Guiltless Grill" favourites and some nutritious sides including veggies, corn on the cob and black beans. The website lists vegetarian options and good nutritional information.

Why choose it? This delicious salad contains half the calories, 60 g less fat and one-third the sodium of the Quesadilla Explosion salad. The honey lime dressing combined with the fruit is outstanding. A way better choice!

→

ALSO CHOOSE

BURGER:
Old Time Burger
› **310** calories
› **65** g fat
  (**20** g saturated)
› **3,230** mg sodium

CHILDREN'S MEAL:
Grilled Chicken Sandwich
› **230** calories
› **5** g fat
  (**0.5** g saturated)
› **440** mg sodium
› **22** g carbohydrates

MEAT:
Classic Sirloin
(not including sides)
› **250** calories
› **7** g fat
  (**3** g saturated)
› **1,580** mg sodium

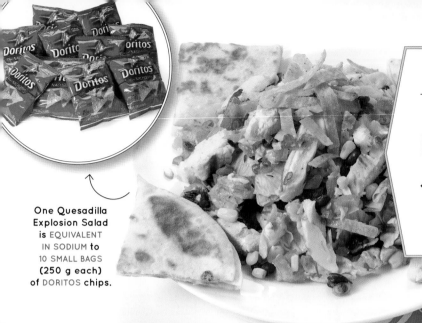

One Quesadilla Explosion Salad is EQUIVALENT IN SODIUM to 10 SMALL BAGS (250 g each) of DORITOS chips.

LOSE IT

QUESADILLA EXPLOSION SALAD
(including balsamic dressing)

1,300 CALORIES
86 G FAT (**28** G SATURATED)
2,470 MG SODIUM

CHILI'S

Why lose it? The word "explosion" in the title can serve as a warning! The cheese topping, combined with the cheese quesadilla wedges and the fried tortilla chips gives you three-quarters of a day's worth of calories, more than a day's worth of fat and saturated fat and over a day's worth of sodium!

ALSO LOSE

BURGER:
Jalapeño Smokehouse Burger
> **2,200** calories
> **144** g fat
  (**46** g saturated)
> **660** mg sodium

CHILDREN'S MEAL:
Grilled Cheese Sandwich
> **530** calories
> **42** g fat
  (**12** g saturated)
> **1,020** mg sodium
> **30** g carbohydrates

MEAT:
Half-Rack of Baby Back Ribs
(not including sides)
> **760** calories
> **49** g fat
  (**20** g saturated)
> **2,590** mg sodium

NUTRITION

Mexican food can be a nutritional disaster if you're not careful about what you order. Foods high in calories, fat and sodium include tortilla chips, taco shells, refried beans, burritos and enchiladas. Stick to the fajitas and vegetable-based dishes.

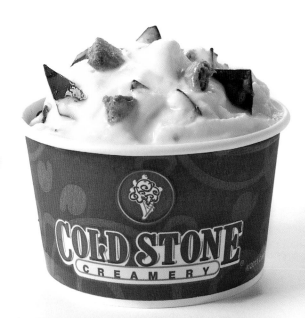

CHOOSE IT

→

CHEESECAKE ICE CREAM

(Love It size, including vanilla wafers, chocolate shavings, Kit Kat mix-ins)

←

780 CALORIES
43 G FAT (**27** G SATURATED)
90 G CARBOHYDRATES
75 G SUGAR

COLD STONE CREAMERY

Cold Stone Creamery opened its doors in 1988 in the U.S. and has expanded to more than 1,400 stores. The chain was introduced to Canada in 2009, in partnership with Tim Hortons. The ice cream is made fresh daily on the premises with high-quality ingredients, and each order is prepared for the customer on a frozen granite stone. The ice cream can be combined with many different mix-ins, which makes the nutritional values on the website difficult to calculate. "Sinless Smoothies" or "Lifestyle Smoothies" are healthier options.

Why choose it? Alone the Love It size Cheesecake Ice Cream, at 520 calories, has about 200 fewer calories than the same size Oreo Ice Cream, at 710 calories. If you pair it with some better-for-you mix-ins, you are saving on calories, fat and sugar. But let's not make this a daily indulgence!

→

ALSO CHOOSE

SMOOTHIES:
Strawberry Bananza
(Love It size)
› **210** calories
› **2** g fat
  (**0** g saturated)
› **54** g carbohydrates
› **32** g sugar

SIGNATURE:
Chocolate Ice Cream
(Love It size)
› **520** calories
› **32** g fat
  (**20** g saturated)
› **53** g carbohydrates
› **48** g sugar

SHAKES:
Cherry Cheeseshake
(Love It size)
› **1,190** calories
› **64** g fat
  (**43** g saturated)
› **146** g carbohydrates
› **107** g sugar

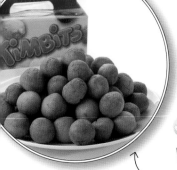

The Oreo ice cream with Reese's Peanut Butter Cups and cookie dough mix-ins has AS MUCH SUGAR as 52 OLD-FASHIONED PLAIN TIMBITS from Tim Hortons.

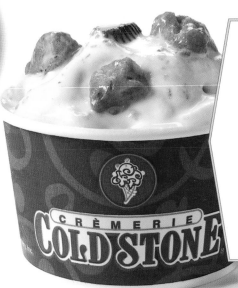

OREO CREME ICE CREAM

(Love It size, including Reese's Peanut Butter Cups, cookie dough mix-ins)

1,080 CALORIES
68 G FAT (**30** G SATURATED)
112 CARBOHYDRATES
104 G SUGAR

COLD STONE CREAMERY

Why lose it? Oreo Ice Cream is an indulgence on its own, but if you add Reese's Peanut Butter Cups and cookie dough to this Love It–size treat you'll be consuming three-quarters of your daily calorie intake, over a day's worth of fat, 3 days' worth of sugar and 1.5 days' worth of carbs (110 g)!

EXERCISE

If you choose the Oreo Ice Cream with Reese's Peanut Butter Cups and cookie dough mix-ins, you'd better be by a swimming pool. You'd have to freestyle swim for two hours to burn off the more than 1,000 calories and 26 tsp (130 mL) of sugar in this treat!

ALSO LOSE

SMOOTHIES:
Mango Pineapple
(Love It size)
› **520** calories
› **5** g fat
   (**4** g saturated)
› **119** g
   carbohydrates
› **88** g sugar

SIGNATURE:
Oreo Ice Cream
(Love It size)
› **710** calories
› **49** g fat
   (**23** g saturated)
› **65** g carbohydrates
› **61** g sugar

SHAKES:
PB&C Shake
(Love It size)
› **1,510** calories
› **103** g fat
   (**54** g saturated)
› **131** g
   carbohydrates
› **117** g sugar

→

BREAKFAST SANDWICH BLT

250 CALORIES
12 G FAT (**5** G SATURATED)
420 MG SODIUM

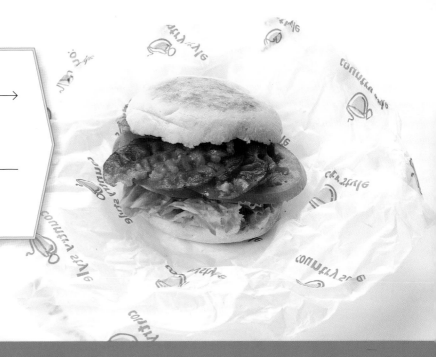

COUNTRY STYLE

Country Style has over 530 locations, mostly in Ontario, and is the second-largest franchisor in that province. It has built its reputation on coffee but also offers fresh baked goods, all-day breakfasts, sandwiches, subs, wraps, salads, soups and chilis. The company is currently promoting itself as a "bistro deli" with a selection of sandwiches that will appeal to the health conscious. The nutritional information available online is well detailed.

Why choose it? You're getting half the calories and less than half the sodium than in the Breakfast Bagel Deluxe. Ask for a slice of cheese rather than the bacon for a healthier protein.

→

ALSO CHOOSE

SIGNATURE SANDWICH:
Assorted Club
› **460** calories
› **16** g fat
  (**5** g saturated)
› **1,370** mg sodium

MUFFINS:
Lemon Cranberry Muffin
› **390** calories
› **16** g fat
  (**2** g saturated)
› **56** g carbohydrates
› **25** g sugar

BEVERAGES:
Iced Cappuccino
› **150** calories
› **3** g fat
  (**0** g saturated)
› **26** g sugar
› **40** mg sodium

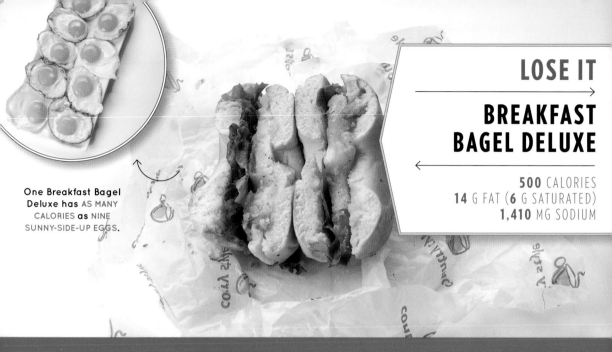

BREAKFAST BAGEL DELUXE

500 CALORIES
14 G FAT (**6** G SATURATED)
1,410 MG SODIUM

One Breakfast Bagel Deluxe has AS MANY CALORIES as NINE SUNNY-SIDE-UP EGGS.

COUNTRY STYLE

Why lose it? This breakfast isn't worth the nutrients since you're getting about one-third of your daily calories and a day's worth of sodium. Almost half the fat is saturated—this comes from the egg, back bacon and cheese.

ALSO LOSE

SIGNATURE SANDWICH:
Spicy Buffalo Chicken Griller
› **630** calories
› **17** g fat
  (**4** g saturated)
› **1,280** mg sodium

MUFFINS:
Corn Muffin
› **480** calories
› **21** g fat
  (**2** g saturated)
› **68** g carbohydrates
› **29** g sugar

BEVERAGES:
Iced Mocha Cappuccino
› **350** calories
› **12** g fat
  (**10** g saturated)
› **390** mg sodium
› **49** g sugar

NUTRITION

Beware of bagels for breakfast. A plain, whole wheat bagel at Country Style has 230 calories and 4 g of fat. A better choice is the toasted English muffin, which has only 140 calories and 1 g of fat.

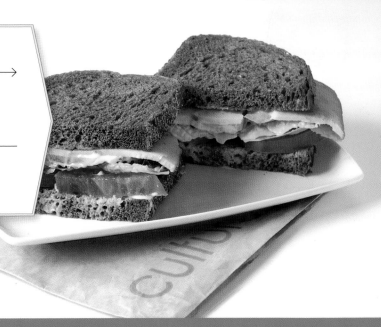

CULTURES

Cultures Restaurant has 55 locations across Canada and was one of the first quick-service restaurants to offer healthy options. Cultures' menu is based on the four S's: salads, sandwiches, soups and smoothies. Everything on the menu is made from scratch. Cultures considers itself to be an ambassador of healthy eating in Canadian food courts, catering to people who understand the connection between longevity and healthy living. The nutrition page on the company website highlights the many menu items that have 5 g of fat or less.

Why choose it? The mayo is just on the bread, not throughout the entire sandwich as with the Egg Club Sandwich. It's even healthier if you ask for mustard instead of mayo.

→

ALSO CHOOSE

SALAD 1:
Asian Chicken Salad
(including Asian sesame dressing, noodles)
› **170** calories
› **10** g fat
  (**1** g saturated)
› **190** mg sodium

SALAD 2:
Tabbouleh
› **130** calories
› **10** g fat
  (**1** g saturated)
› **260** mg sodium

WRAP:
Turkey Wrap
› **320** calories
› **6** g fat
  (**1** g saturated)
› **780** mg sodium

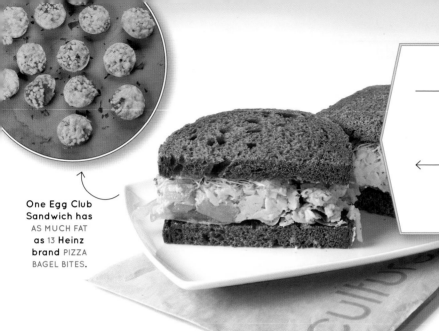

One Egg Club Sandwich has AS MUCH FAT as 13 **Heinz** brand PIZZA BAGEL BITES.

CULTURES

Why lose it? Eggs may be healthy on their own (though higher in calories, fat and saturated fat than turkey breast), but mayonnaise adds to the calories and fat.

ALSO LOSE

SALAD 1:
Bean Salad
> **410** calories
> **23** g fat
  (**2** g saturated)
> **970** mg sodium

SALAD 2:
Orzo Salad
(including Greek dressing)
> **270** calories
> **17** g fat
  (**4** g saturated)
> **1,050** mg sodium

WRAPS:
Tuna Wrap
> **430** calories
> **17** g fat
  (**4** g saturated)
> **700** mg sodium

NUTRITION

Eggs are a healthy protein; each one contains approximately 70 calories, 5 g of fat, 200 mg of cholesterol and 6 g of protein. A typical egg salad sandwich has two to three eggs, so consuming one of these daily might be too much for those with heart or cholesterol issues. Natural egg substitutes, such as Break Free, contain a liquid mixture comprised of 80 percent egg whites and 20 percent egg yolks. One serving of Break Free contains only 40 calories, 1 g of fat, 35 mg of cholesterol and 6 g of protein. A much healthier choice, and it also tastes great!

→

CHOCOLATE CONE
(medium, 199 g)

←

360 CALORIES
10 G FAT (**6** G SATURATED)
59 G CARBOHYDRATES
40 G SUGAR

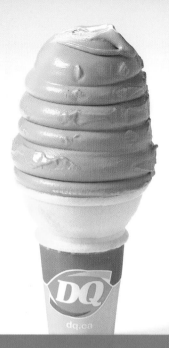

DAIRY QUEEN

Dairy Queen first opened in 1940 in Joliet, Illinois. Today, it has more than 5,700 stores in 19 countries, primarily in the United States and Canada. The first Dairy Queen in Canada opened in Saskatchewan, and the busiest Canadian location is in Charlottetown, Prince Edward Island. DQ has many frozen treats, as well as savoury fast-food items. For those watching their calories and fat, DQ now offers Mini Blizzards and soft frozen yogurt. Nutritionals are available online, but read carefully because the various sizes and large number of offerings can be tricky to navigate.

Why choose it? Just eliminating the chocolate coating of the Chocolate Dipped Cone reduces the calories considerably and cuts the fat and saturated fat by more than half.

ALSO CHOOSE

BLIZZARD:
Mint Oreo Blizzard
(medium, 334 g)
› **680** calories
› **25** g fat
  (**17** g saturated)
› **79** g sugar

BASKET:
Chicken Strip Basket
(396 g, including sauce, french fries, 4 pieces of chicken)
› **790** calories
› **36** g fat
  (**3** g saturated)
› **2,050** mg sodium

BURGER:
Cheeseburger
› **400** calories
› **19** g fat
  (**8** g saturated)
› **880** mg sodium

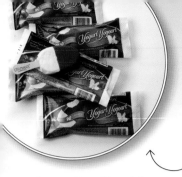

One medium Chocolate
Dipped Cone has
AS MUCH FAT **as** FIVE
Chapman's VANILLA FROZEN
YOGURT BARS.

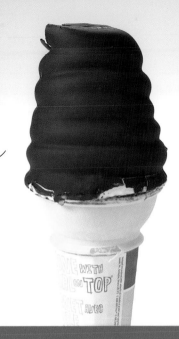

CHOCOLATE
DIPPED CONE
(medium, 199 g)

470 CALORIES
21 G FAT (**16** G SATURATED)
63 G CARBOHYDRATES
46 G SUGAR

DAIRY QUEEN

Why lose it? The chocolate dip adds an extra 100 calories, doubles the fat and more than doubles the saturated fat! Plus, the dip is made from a chocolate compound, so you're not even getting all those yummy chocolate antioxidants!

ALSO LOSE

BLIZZARD:
**Turtle Pecan
Cluster Blizzard**
(medium, 334 g)
› **1,030** calories
› **53** g fat
 (**26** g saturated)
› **115** g sugar

BASKET:
Poutine Basket
(11 oz/528 g,
including gravy,
cheese curds)
› **1,240** calories
› **66** g fat
 (**22** g saturated)
› **2,760** mg sodium

BURGER:
**Crispy Flame
Thrower Chicken
Sandwich**
› **820** calories
› **53** g fat
 (**10** g saturated)
› **2,180** mg sodium

EXERCISE

Every time you indulge at Dairy Queen, consider walking to the restaurant and back home. To burn off the medium Chocolate Dipped Cone you'll need to briskly walk at 6 km per hour for about 1.5 hours. Indulge occasionally, or cut back on your next meal.

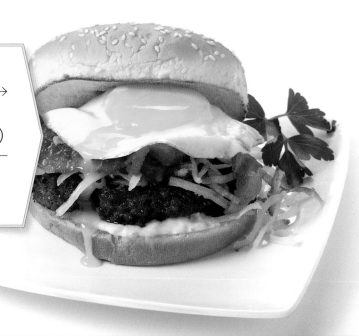

CHOOSE IT

→

SLAMBURGER
(9 oz/255 g, including cheese sauce)

750 CALORIES
60 G FAT (**24** G SATURATED)
1,560 MG SODIUM

DENNY'S

With over 1,500 locations in North America, Denny's has been serving good food at great value for over 50 years. Denny's is a large, full-service family restaurant chain with 49 locations in Canada. It was originally known for breakfasts, but the lunch and dinner menus, which include a wide variety of salads, soups, sandwiches and burgers, are also very popular. Nutritionals are detailed on the website, but the information is often incomplete. Salad info often doesn't include dressing, and entrée info doesn't include sides, which means you have to do the math!

Why choose it? The Slamburger sounds indulgent, but it actually has less fat and close to half the calories and sodium of the Western Burger. The hash browns are grilled, compared with the Western Burger's fried onion rings, and the bacon and egg don't count for as many calories as the Western Burger's extra melted cheese.

→

ALSO CHOOSE

SPECIALTY SANDWICH:
The Super Bird
(10 oz/283 g)
› **560** calories
› **27** g fat
  (**8** g saturated)
› **2,360** mg sodium

SIDES:
Hash Browns
(5 oz/142 g)
› **210** calories
› **12** g fat
  (**3** g saturated)
› **650** mg sodium

APPETIZERS:
Chicken Wings
(8 oz/227 g, including buffalo sauce)
› **300** calories
› **21** g fat
  (**5** g saturated)
› **1,940** mg sodium

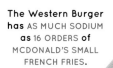

The Western Burger has AS MUCH SODIUM as 16 ORDERS of MCDONALD'S SMALL FRENCH FRIES.

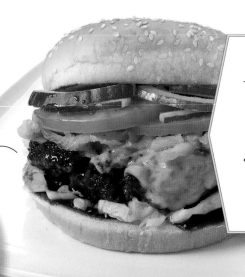

WESTERN BURGER

(17 oz/482 g, including tangy steak sauce)

1,300 CALORIES
82 G FAT (**30** G SATURATED)
2,700 MG SODIUM

DENNY'S

Why lose it? The Western Burger looks more innocent than the Slamburger, but the Onion Tanglers (onion rings) are breaded and deep-fried, there's excess cheese and the tangy steak sauce is sugar based.

ALSO LOSE

SPECIALTY SANDWICH:
Chicken Sandwich
(15 oz/425 g, including honey mustard dressing)
› **1,190** calories
› **65** g fat
  (**11** g saturated)
› **2,910** mg sodium

SIDES:
Onion Rings
(5 oz/142 g)
› **520** calories
› **36** g fat
  (**2** g saturated)
› **980** mg sodium

APPETIZERS:
Smothered Cheese Fries
(10 oz/283 g, including ranch dressing)
› **870** calories
› **52** g fat
  (**18** g saturated)
› **1,240** mg sodium

WEIGHT LOSS

By losing the Western Burger and choosing the Slamburger once a week for a year, you can easily drop 8 lb (4 kg) without changing anything else in your diet or lifestyle. That's about one and a half dress sizes!

CHOOSE IT

→

MAKE YOUR OWN
(two medium slices, thin crust, marinara sauce, cheese, pineapple, ham)

←

314 CALORIES
15 G FAT (**6** G SATURATED)
690 MG SODIUM
30 G CARBOHYDRATES

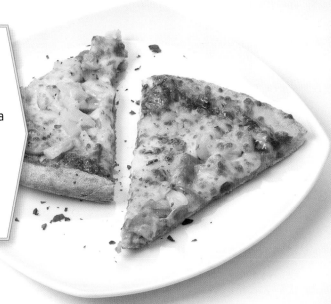

DOMINO'S PIZZA

Domino's has been making pizza since 1960 and is the largest pizza chain in the world, with over 9,000 outlets in 60 countries. The first Domino's to open outside the United States was in Winnipeg in 1983. Pizza speciality crusts include traditional hand tossed, thin crust, deep-dish and Brooklyn. Lighter option crusts are now available. Determining the nutritional information for your pizza online can be challenging because of all the choices in crusts, toppings and sizes.

Why choose it? The thin crust is crisp and delicious and saves you a whopping amount of empty calories and fat, even with the cheese and ham toppings. All nutritional information listed is based on two slices of a 12 inch (30 cm) medium-size pizza, each slice being about one-eighth of the whole pizza.

ALSO CHOOSE

→

SAUCE:
Marinara
› **15** calories
› **0** g fat
› **108** mg sodium

PIZZA CRUST:
Thin Crust
› **168** calories
› **7** g fat
› **30** mg sodium
› **23** g carbohydrates

TOPPINGS:
Ham
› **23** calories
› **1** g fat
› **255** mg sodium

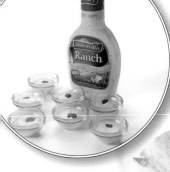

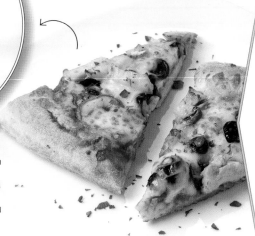

Two slices of deep-dish pizza with marinara sauce, extra cheese, chicken and black olives is EQUIVALENT IN FAT to 7 TBSP (105 mL) of HIDDEN VALLEY LIGHT RANCH DRESSING.

LOSE IT

→

MAKE YOUR OWN
(two medium slices, deep-dish crust, marinara sauce, extra cheese, chicken, mushrooms, black olives)

←

560 CALORIES
26 G FAT (**10** G SATURATED)
1,470 MG SODIUM
58 G CARBOHYDRATES

DOMINO'S PIZZA

Why lose it? Beware of the words "deep-dish," a thick, oily pizza crust that acts as a large bowl whose edges are higher than the filling. This crust adds calories, and the extra cheese adds calories, fat and sodium. You're getting one-third of your daily calories, half your daily fat and a day's worth of sodium.

ALSO LOSE

SAUCE:
Garlic Parmesan
> **98** calories
> **10** g fat
> **170** mg sodium

PIZZA CRUST:
Deep-Dish Crust
> **322** calories
> **11** g fat
> **504** mg sodium
> **50** g carbohydrates

TOPPINGS:
Italian Sausage
> **88** calories
> **8** g fat
> **258** mg sodium

FOOD TRIVIA

Domino's delivers over 400 million pizzas a year throughout North America. That's a pizza and an extra slice for every man, woman and child and more than one million pizzas a day! In the United States, Domino's drivers cover over nine million miles (14 million km) each week, or 37 trips to the moon!

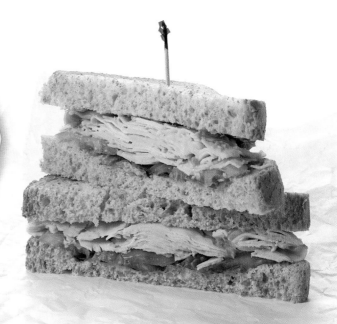

CHOOSE IT

TURKEY BREAST SANDWICH

303 CALORIES
3 G FAT (**0.3** G SATURATED)
1,035 MG SODIUM

DRUXY'S

Druxy's opened its doors in 1976 in Toronto, and has since expanded throughout Canada and the U.S. Originally known for its premium smoked meat and Old World deli flavours, Druxy's has recently repositioned itself to keep up with health trends. This diner serves classic and nouveau deli sandwiches, soups, salads and breakfasts. The menu accommodates special diets, featuring gluten-free, lactose-free and vegan options. The nutritionals can be found online; the Heart and Stroke Foundation approves the highlighted items on the menu.

Why choose it? The turkey breast is roasted, not smoked, which cuts down the sodium. As well, it doesn't have the fat of pastrami, meaning significantly fewer calories and less fat.

ALSO CHOOSE

SANDWICH:
Turkey Club
› **274** calories
› **4** g fat
  (**1** g saturated)
› **878** mg sodium

SALAD:
Greek Feta Pasta Salad
(200 g)
› **360** calories
› **22** g fat
  (**3** g saturated)
› **620** mg sodium

SOUP:
Beef Noodle Soup
› **100** calories
› **2** g fat
› **600** mg sodium

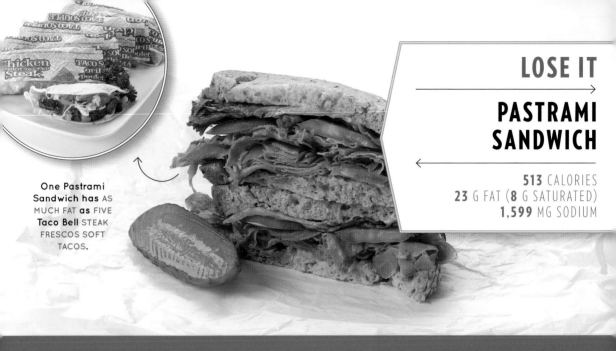

PASTRAMI SANDWICH

513 CALORIES
23 G FAT (**8** G SATURATED)
1,599 MG SODIUM

One Pastrami Sandwich has AS MUCH FAT as FIVE **Taco Bell** STEAK FRESCOS SOFT TACOS.

DRUXY'S

Why lose it? Pastrami is smoked corned beef, which is beef marinated in a brine, a salty preservative. This translates into excess salt and unhealthy nitrites and nitrates. This sandwich has more calories and about eight times the fat of the Turkey Breast Sandwich, not to mention the day's worth of sodium!

ALSO LOSE

SANDWICH:
Reuben Sandwich
› **591** calories
› **27** g fat
   (**13** g saturated)
› **1,783** mg sodium

SALAD:
Wheat Berry Salad
(200 g)
› **500** calories
› **36** g fat
   (**3** g saturated)
› **400** mg sodium

SOUP:
Tomato Red Bisque
› **350** calories
› **24** g fat
› **970** mg sodium

HEALTH WARNING

Pastrami is a spiced, cured meat that was originally produced to stay fresh for weeks. Salt and nitrites are added for colour and flavour. For 113 g of pastrami you're having about 170 calories, 7 g of fat (half of which is saturated), 100 mg of cholesterol and over 1,000 mg of sodium. Eating cured meats regularly will increase your risk for developing heart disease, high blood pressure, cholesterol and certain cancers.

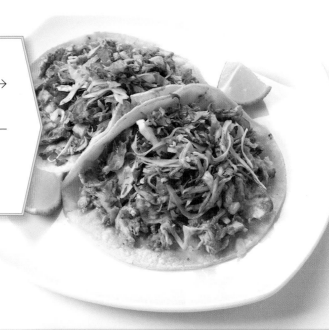

CHOOSE IT

→

LOS CABOS

←

484 CALORIES
24 G FAT (**10** G SATURATED)
1,208 MG SODIUM
20 G CARBOHYDRATES

EARLS

Earls is a family restaurant established in 1982 by Leroy Earl Fuller and his son, Stanley Earl Fuller. With its West Coast flair, Earls has expanded from a laid-back "beer and burger joint" to a comfortable, affordable restaurant with an upscale atmosphere. The dishes are inspired by popular cuisines and range from unique appetizers and salads to sustainable varieties of fish, Angus beef, pastas and sandwiches. Earls now has over 50 restaurants throughout Canada and the U.S. Nutritional information can be found on the restaurant website under the menu tab.

Why choose it? With grilled chicken and corn tortillas, which are lower in calories, fat and sodium than flour tortillas, the calories and fat in this meal are about half those of the Chili Chicken even with the two cheeses and avocado corn salsa.

→

ALSO CHOOSE

PIZZA:
Naples Margherita
(362 g)
› **748** calories
› **25** g fat
  (**10** g saturated)
› **1,655** mg sodium

MEAT:
Certified Angus Beef Top Sirloin
(9 oz/255 g, including mashed potato, vegetables)
› **848** calories
› **52** g fat
  (**27** g saturated)
› **3,498** mg sodium

PASTA:
Lobster Gnocchi
› **892** calories
› **43** g fat
  (**21** g saturated)
› **2,253** mg sodium

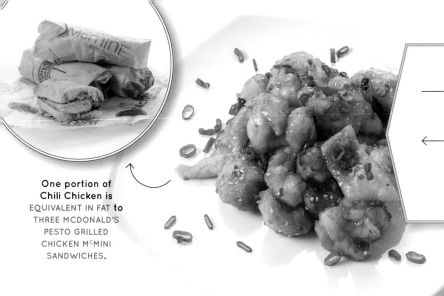

LOSE IT

CHILI CHICKEN

1,015 CALORIES
41 G FAT (**4** G SATURATED)
779 MG SODIUM
125 G CARBOHYDRATES

One portion of Chili Chicken is EQUIVALENT IN FAT to THREE MCDONALD'S PESTO GRILLED CHICKEN McMINI SANDWICHES.

EARLS

Why lose it? The breaded and fried chicken, fried wontons and sweet sauce are the main reasons to lose this meal, which gives you about three-quarters of your day's calories and fat and about half your day's carbohydrates.

ALSO LOSE

PIZZA:
California Prawn Pesto
(470 g)
› **1,137** calories
› **51** g fat
   (**24** g saturated)
› **2,100** mg sodium

MEAT:
BBQ Back Ribs
(including potato salad, coleslaw)
› **1,164** calories
› **78** g fat
   (**28** g saturated)
› **2,958** mg sodium

PASTA:
Dungness Crab & Asparagus Linguini
› **1,193** calories
› **82** g fat
   (**29** g saturated)
› **1,415** mg sodium

HEALTH WARNING

In general, the entire menu at Earls is high in calories, fat and sodium. Many of the dishes are close to an entire day's worth of calories and sodium. For an appetizer, try a non-cream-based soup (still high in sodium), or a side salad with dressing on the side. Stick to steaks or fish for your main course.

CHOOSE IT

CHICKEN PARMIGIANA SANDWICH

560 CALORIES
15 G FAT (**5** G SATURATED)
2,210 MG SODIUM

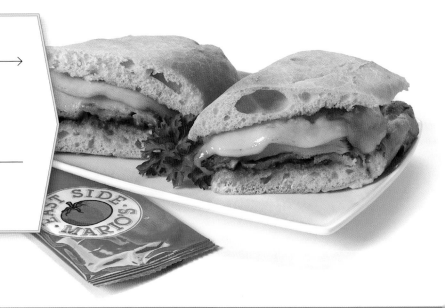

EAST SIDE MARIO'S

East Side Mario's has over 100 locations in Canada as well as some in the United States. A casual dining restaurant, it features Italian-American cuisine and is marketed as "a taste of Italy." East Side Mario's is managed by Prime Restaurants, which also operates Pat and Mario's, Casey's and The Bier Markt. The website includes nutritional information, but there is no evidence of a healthier menu initiative to date.

Why choose it? The chicken breast is baked, and even with the addition of mozzarella cheese, Napolitana sauce and a bun it has 250 fewer calories and 30 g less fat than the Tuscan Turkey Club.

ALSO CHOOSE

CLASSIC ENTRÉE:
Mario's Chicken Parmigiana
(including fettuccine alfredo side)
› **820** calories
› **22** g fat
  (**10** g saturated)
› **2,210** mg sodium

CHILDREN'S MENU:
Kid's Cheese Cappelletti
› **460** calories
› **15** g fat
  (**8** g saturated)
› **1,030** mg sodium

SIDES:
Spaghettini with Herbed Olive Oil
› **260** calories
› **2** g fat
  (**0** g saturated)
› **260** mg sodium

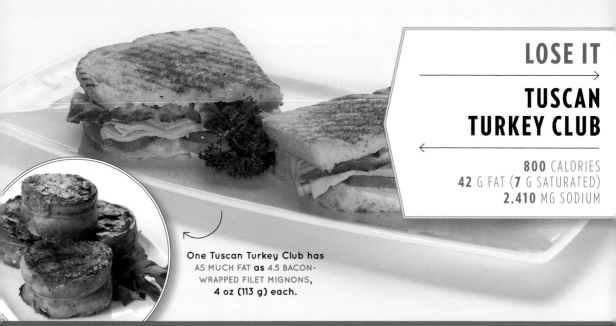

One Tuscan Turkey Club has
AS MUCH FAT **as** 4.5 BACON-
WRAPPED FILET MIGNONS,
4 oz (113 g) each.

EAST SIDE MARIO'S

Why lose it? The turkey club sandwich has high-calorie bacon and mayonnaise. The Tuscan bread adds to the calories and fat.

NUTRITION

Any clubhouse tends to be high in calories, fat and sodium. It consists of three slices of bread, chicken or turkey, bacon and cheese, and is slathered with mayonnaise. Not a "light" meal.

ALSO LOSE

CLASSIC ENTRÉE:
Linguine Chicken Amatriciana
› **1,070** calories
› **54** g fat
  (**11** g saturated)
› **1,650** mg sodium

CHILDREN'S MENU:
Mac 'n' Cheese Bites
› **530** calories
› **27** g fat
  (**7** g saturated)
› **1,880** mg sodium

SIDES:
Mario Potatoes
› **770** calories
› **57** g fat
  (**11** g saturated)
› **450** mg sodium

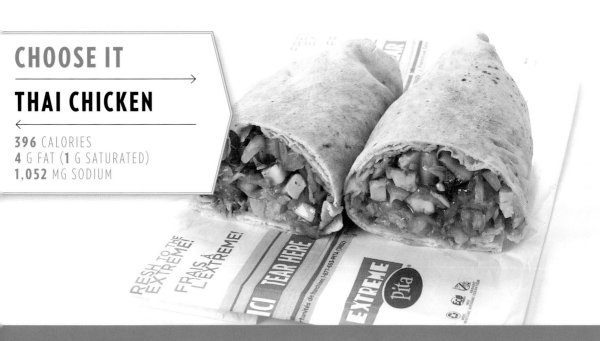

EXTREME PITA

Extreme Pita was established in 1997 and now has over 200 locations in Canada and the United States. It was started by two brothers, Alex and Mark Rechichi, who realized that nutritious and versatile pita bread could be used as a wrap and was strong enough to hold an array of ingredients. Extreme Pita's commitment to health is evident in the number of items on its menu that bear the Health Check, a sign of approval by the Heart and Stroke Foundation. The website includes a nutritional guide and a gluten-free menu.

Why choose it? The Thai Chicken dish is packed with low-calorie veggies, and the chili sauce only adds 55 calories and no fat. All the nutritional information is for a regular-size pita (417 g).

ALSO CHOOSE

FREESTYLE PITA 1:
Philly Cheese Steak
› **527** calories
› **19** g fat
  (**7** g saturated)
› **1,088** mg sodium

FREESTYLE PITA 2:
Club Pita with Turkey, Ham and Bacon
› **400** calories
› **9** g fat
  (**3** g saturated)
› **1,712** mg sodium

CHEF-INSPIRED PITA:
Chicken Caesar
› **486** calories
› **13** g fat
  (**4** g saturated)
› **1,550** mg sodium

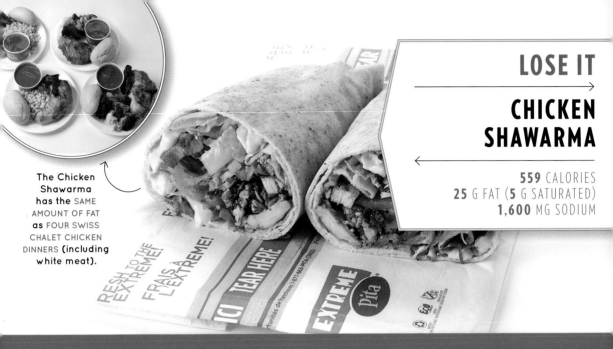

The Chicken Shawarma has the SAME AMOUNT OF FAT as FOUR SWISS CHALET CHICKEN DINNERS (including white meat).

LOSE IT

CHICKEN SHAWARMA

559 CALORIES
25 G FAT (**5** G SATURATED)
1,600 MG SODIUM

EXTREME PITA

Why lose it? It's not the chicken adding to the calories and fat, but the lemon-garlic shawarma sauce, which adds an extra 140 calories and 14 g of fat!

ALSO LOSE

FREESTYLE PITA 1:
Chipotle Steak
› **658** calories
› **34** g fat
  (**4** g saturated)
› **1,535** mg sodium

FREESTYLE PITA 2:
Gyro Pita
› **621** calories
› **32** g fat
  (**8** g saturated)
› **1,274** mg sodium

CHEF-INSPIRED PITA:
Chicken Souvlaki
› **615** calories
› **29** g fat
  (**10** g saturated)
› **1,676** mg sodium

FOOD FACT

Shawarma is the fast food of the Middle East and is now very popular in the West. It can be either shaved lamb, chicken or turkey. The meat is placed on a spit and grilled for up to a day. It can be served with hummus or a higher-fat, oil-based sauce. It's made by stacking strips of fat and seasoned pieces of meat alternately on a stick; the meat slowly roasts as the spit turns, and is then shaved into thin slices for sandwiches.

CHOOSE IT

WRAP
(whole wheat tortilla, diced tomatoes, goat cheese, turkey, salsa)

262 CALORIES
11 G FAT (**3** G SATURATED)
1,077 MG SODIUM
57 G CARBOHYDRATES

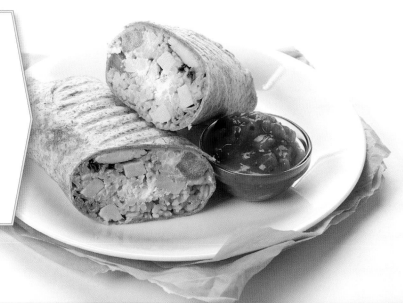

FRESHII

Freshii was founded in 2005 in Toronto by a young man named Matthew Corrin, who had a vision of offering fresh, healthy, custom-made food and fast service. Originally called Lettuce Eatery, it opened to long lines and sold out of food after one lunch hour! Freshii is now known for its convenience and choice of fresh meals and snacks served in an environmentally sustainable setting. The online menu has a nutritional calculator but you have to be organized to get the correct numbers.

Why choose it? Roasted turkey is lean, and there are enough carbs in the tortillas, so you don't need to add rice. The salsa is virtually calorie and fat free compared with the creamy ranch dressing in the "Lose It" burrito.

ALSO CHOOSE

BREAKFAST WRAP:
Spinach & Goat Cheese Wrap
(including roasted red peppers, mushrooms, Dijonnaise)
› **182** calories
› **5** g fat
  (**2** g saturated)
› **342** mg sodium

SALAD:
Romaine
(including turkey, avocado, tomato, jack and cheddar cheeses, low-fat ranch dressing)
› **385** calories
› **28** g fat
  (**8** g saturated)
› **1,108** mg sodium

BOWL:
Teriyaki Chicken Bowl
(including brown rice, vegetables, teriyaki sauce)
› **391** calories
› **2** g fat
  (**0** g saturated)
› **605** mg sodium

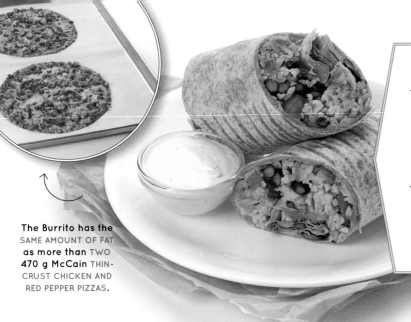

LOSE IT

BURRITO

(whole wheat tortilla brown rice, black beans, steak, jack and cheddar cheeses, avocado, ranch dressing)

1,036 CALORIES
60 G FAT (**15** G SATURATED)
1315 MG SODIUM
130 G CARBOHYDRATES

The Burrito has the SAME AMOUNT OF FAT as more than TWO 470 g McCain THIN-CRUST CHICKEN AND RED PEPPER PIZZAS.

FRESHII

Why lose it? The brown rice and whole wheat tortilla are healthier than their white flour counterparts, but you don't need both. The steak has more calories and fat than turkey. Avocadoes are heart healthy, but add calories and fat, as do the cheeses and dressing.

ALSO LOSE

BREAKFAST WRAP:
Bacon & Egg Wrap
(including smoked bacon, jack and cheddar cheeses, Dijonaise)
› **312** calories
› **14** g fat
  (**5** g saturated)
› **653** mg sodium

SALAD:
Spinach
(including roast chicken, chopped dates, walnuts, feta, croutons)
› **555** calories
› **31** g fat
  (**14** g saturated)
› **965** mg sodium

BOWL:
Bliss Bowl
(including brown rice, double avocado, roasted red pepper, tomato, goat cheese, olive oil)
› **424** calories
› **11** g fat
  (**3** g saturated)
› **73** mg sodium

WEIGHT LOSS

We've been taught to believe that anything we order at a salad establishment, even sandwiches or wraps, must be healthy. But here you can see that there is an enormous difference in calories and fat between a burrito and a wrap. If you enjoy eating the burrito rather than the wrap a couple of times per week, you may see a 22 lb (11 kg) weight gain at the end of the year!

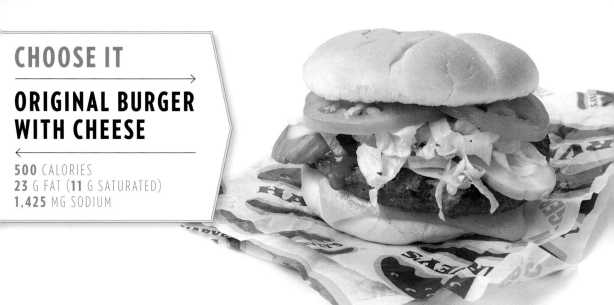

CHOOSE IT

→

ORIGINAL BURGER WITH CHEESE

←

500 CALORIES
23 G FAT (**11** G SATURATED)
1,425 MG SODIUM

HARVEY'S

Harvey's opened its first restaurant in 1959 just north of Toronto. Today, with over 286 locations across Canada, Harvey's is still making hamburgers a "beautiful thing." The chain is owned by Cara Operations and is the second-largest Canadian restaurant chain. It is known for its beef burgers charbroiled on a flame grill. It also offers chicken and veggie burgers and classic sides. The children's menu consists of the basic hamburgers, hot dogs and fries and lacks healthy options. The website has nutritional information as well as an allergy listing.

Why choose it? A good old beef burger is healthier than the Crispy Chicken Burger. Just add loads of veggies and non-fat condiments, and you will save over 220 calories and 16 g of fat.

→

ALSO CHOOSE

SNACKS:
Li'l Original Hamburger
(including cheese, bacon)
› **260** calories
› **12** g fat
  (**6** g saturated)
› **680** mg sodium

SIDES:
Fries
(large, 150 g)
› **410** calories
› **16** g fat
  (**1** g saturated)
› **1,190** mg sodium

DIPPING SAUCE:
Sweet 'n' Sour Sauce
› **80** calories
› **0.5** g fat
  (**0** g saturated)

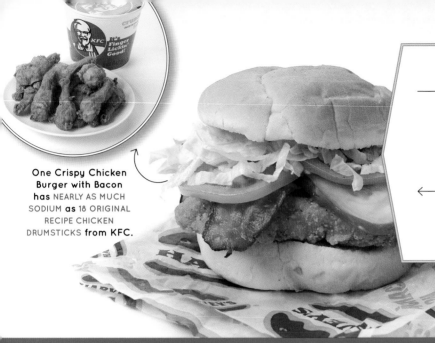

One Crispy Chicken Burger with Bacon **has** NEARLY AS MUCH SODIUM **as** 18 ORIGINAL RECIPE CHICKEN DRUMSTICKS **from KFC.**

LOSE IT

CRISPY CHICKEN BURGER WITH BACON

724 CALORIES
39 G FAT (**5** G SATURATED)
2,098 MG SODIUM

HARVEY'S

Why lose it? We think a chicken burger is healthier than beef, but not when the chicken is breaded and deep-fried. Add mayo, spicy mesquite sauce and bacon, and you're consuming half your daily calories, more than three-quarters of your daily fat and more than a day's worth of sodium.

NUTRITION

When choosing toppings for any burger, keep in mind that mustard, ketchup, A1 sauce, barbeque sauce, vegetables and relish are all low-calorie and low-fat topping choices. Avoid or limit toppings like cheese, bacon, mayonnaise and "special" sauces (which usually contain oil or mayo).

ALSO LOSE

SNACKS:
Bacon Cheddar Dog
(including ketchup, relish)
› **440** calories
› **21** g fat
   (**10** g saturated)
› **1,210** mg sodium

SIDES:
Onion Rings
(large, 144 g)
› **550** calories
› **29** g fat
   (**3** g saturated)
› **1,580** mg sodium

DIPPING SAUCE:
Honey Mustard
› **160** calories
› **12** g fat
   (**2** g saturated)

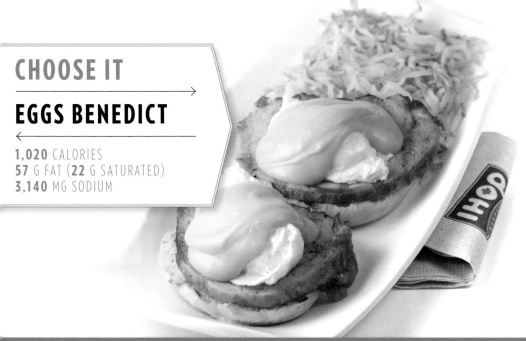

CHOOSE IT

→

EGGS BENEDICT

←

1,020 CALORIES
57 G FAT (**22** G SATURATED)
3,140 MG SODIUM

IHOP

IHOP (International House of Pancakes) has over 1,500 franchises throughout North and Central America and the Caribbean. It is known for its signature pancakes, omelettes and other breakfast specialities, but it also offers a wide variety of lunch, dinner and snack items. With respect to healthy menu items, IHOP offers a "Simple & Fit" under-600-calorie menu and gives tips on how to enjoy lower-calorie versions of traditional IHOP menu items by making a few changes when you order.

Why choose it? The eggs are poached not fried, and the ham has fewer calories and less fat than fried steak. If you ask for the hollandaise on the side adding just a couple of tablespoons you will save calories and fat as well.

→

ALSO CHOOSE

OMELETTE:
Make Your Own
(including provolone, ham, vegetables)
› **650** calories
› **45** g fat
  (**17** g saturated)
› **1,200** mg sodium

SALAD:
Chicken Fajita Salad
› **790** calories
› **44** g fat
  (**21** g saturated)
› **1,600** mg sodium

APPETIZERS:
Monster Mozza Sticks
› **770** calories
› **38** g fat
  (**16** g saturated)
› **2,680** mg sodium

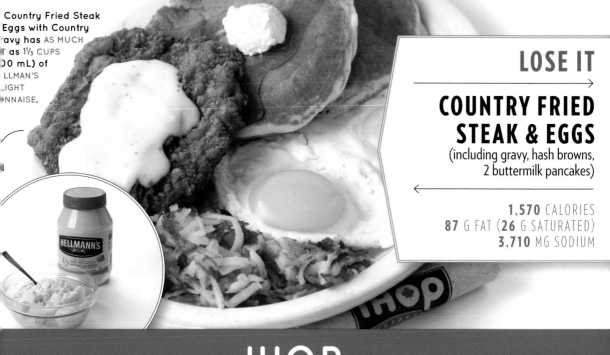

Country Fried Steak Eggs with Country Gravy has AS MUCH T as 1⅓ CUPS 0 mL) of LLMAN'S IGHT NNAISE.

LOSE IT

COUNTRY FRIED STEAK & EGGS
(including gravy, hash browns, 2 buttermilk pancakes)

1,570 CALORIES
87 G FAT (**26** G SATURATED)
3,710 MG SODIUM

IHOP

Why lose it? The number of words in this description should warn you that this is a once-a-year meal! Fried eggs, fried beef steak and country gravy tells you where a day's worth of calories and fat and two days' worth of sodium are coming from. This should be an easy one to lose!

ALSO LOSE

OMELETTE:
Make Your Own
(including cheddar, sausage, tomatoes, green peppers, onions)
› **960** calories
› **72** g fat
  (**29** g saturated)
› **1,230** mg sodium

SALAD:
Grilled Chicken Caesar Salad
› **1,050** calories
› **75** g fat
  (**16** g saturated)
› **2,120** mg sodium

APPETIZERS:
Onion Rings
› **1,250** calories
› **69** g fat
  (**12** g saturated)
› **1,110** mg sodium

MENU

In 11 pages of nutritional information on IHOP meals, it's not easy to find a lot of healthy items, except for those on the "Simple & Fit" menu. Most of the omelettes are around 900 calories, with 60 g of fat and 2,000 mg of sodium, over three-quarters of a day's worth of calories and a full day's worth of fat and sodium. Avoid the combos, which are around 1,500 calories, 70 g of fat and 3,000 mg of sodium! Your best bets are the French toast, waffles and pancakes without the butter or whipped cream.

CHOOSE IT

ROASTED GARLIC BRUSCHETTA

690 CALORIES
23 G FAT (**5** G SATURATED)
1,538 MG SODIUM

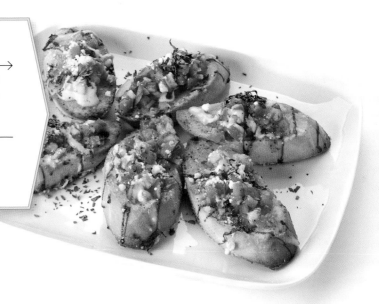

PART 1 JACK ASTOR'S

Jack Astor's opened its doors in 1990 and now has 32 restaurants across Ontario, Quebec, Nova Scotia, Alberta and now New York. Its laid-back environment is perfect for family meals, snacks with coworkers, and nights out with friends. There's even a high-energy late-night bar scene. Menu items vary from classic burgers, fries and sandwiches to steaks, hand-tossed pizzas and ethnic favourites like pad Thai and fresh Greek salad. Jack Astor's nutritional information is among the most detailed I've come

Why choose it? There's nothing deep-fried here. If you're sharing, this tasty appetizer (with Parmesan cheeses, aioli and glaze) is one you don't need to feel guilty about. It has a third of the calories and sodium, one-sixth of the fat and less than one-tenth of the saturated fat of Jack's Ultimate Nachos.

ALSO CHOOSE

APPETIZER:
Summer Rolls
(including chicken, vegetables, noodles, sauce)
> **492** calories
> **5** g fat (**0.4** g saturated)
> **54** g sugar
> **3,416** mg sodium

SANDWICH:
Le Montreal Special
(including smoked beef, smoked mozzarella)
> **337** calories
> **10** g fat (**6** g saturated)
> **1,299** mg sodium

DINNER:
Indian Butter Chicken
(including basmati rice, naan bread)
> **1,033** calories
> **34** g fat (**13** g saturated)
> **1,893** mg sodium

continued on page 66

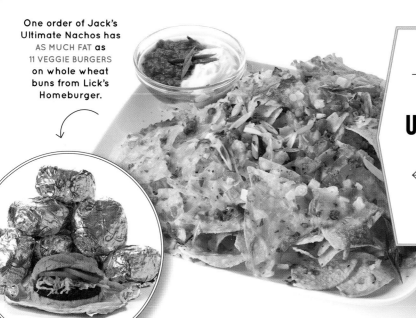

One order of Jack's Ultimate Nachos has AS MUCH FAT as 11 VEGGIE BURGERS on whole wheat buns from Lick's Homeburger.

JACK'S ULTIMATE NACHOS, VEGETARIAN

2,485 CALORIES
140 G FAT (**57** G SATURATED)
4,495 MG SODIUM

JACK ASTOR'S PART 1

Why lose it? This appetizer spells trouble! The tortillas, cheeses, sour cream and salsa, add up to 1½ days calories, two days of fat and almost three days of saturated fat and sodium. You'll be lucky if you make it out of the restaurant!

ALSO LOSE

APPETIZER:
Bangkok Spring Rolls
(including noodles, vegetables, sauce)
> **1,142** calories
> **61** g fat
   (**6** g saturated)
> **85** g sugar
> **2,015** mg sodium

SANDWICH:
Jack's Veggie Burger
(including barbecue sauce, roasted mushrooms, cheddar cheese, chipotle mayo)
> **805** calories
> **43** g fat
   (**13** g saturated)
> **1,772** mg sodium

DINNER:
Parmesan Chicken Bowtie Pasta
(including Asiago cheese, cheese sauce, sundried tomatoes)
> **1,473** calories
> **72** g fat
   (**38** g saturated)
> **3,077** mg sodium

HEALTH WARNING

If you're ordering nachos, just remember that most tortilla chips are deep-fried, and 10 chips have about 150 calories and 7 g of fat. Baked tortilla chips have 129 calories and 4 g of fat. Sour cream contains 14 percent milk fat, and one-quarter of a cup has 120 calories, 12 g of fat and 7.4 g of saturated fat. Use light sour cream at home and save half the calories and fat.

CHOOSE IT

→

CALIFORNIA GRILLED CHICKEN SALAD
(with balsamic dressing)

←

264 CALORIES
8 G FAT (**1** G SATURATED)
510 MG SODIUM

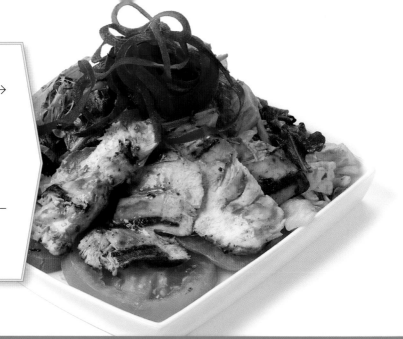

PART 2 JACK ASTOR'S

continued from page 64

across. It includes allergy information for each item as well as gluten-free choices and tips for lowering sodium. Yet many of Jack Astor's items are very high in sodium, so look carefully at the nutritionals before you order. If you want to eat healthy, check out the SFL (Simply For Life) menu. The SFL program actually includes nutritional consultants who are available to speak with customers about their dietary needs. What an innovative idea!

Why choose it? With nothing fried and only pine nuts as a garnish, this dish has 613 fewer calories than the Asian Chicken Salad, as well as 22 g less fat and 2,546 mg less sodium! The balsamic glaze is very low in calories and virtually fat free.

→

ALSO CHOOSE

STEAK DINNER:
Butter Brushed Sirloin Steak
› **335** calories
› **20** g fat
  (**10** g saturated)
› **203** mg sodium

CHILDREN'S MEAL:
Pepperoni Pizza
› **319** calories
› **18** g fat
  (**7** g saturated)
› **849** mg sodium

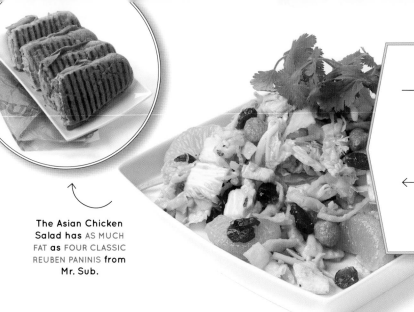

LOSE IT

ASIAN CHICKEN SALAD
(with sesame soy dressing)

877 CALORIES
30 G FAT (**2.3** G SATURATED)
3,056 MG SODIUM

JACK ASTOR'S PART 2

Why lose it? The roasted chicken breast and the napa cabbage, sundried cranberries and mandarin oranges are all healthy. What puts this salad into the higher calorie and fat category is the peanuts, fried wonton crisps and oil-based sesame soy dressing. This is more than half your daily calories and fat and two days' worth of sodium.

ALSO LOSE

STEAK DINNER:
Jack's
Chicago Steak
› **687** calories
› **50** g fat
(**32** g saturated)
› **322** mg sodium

CHILDREN'S MEAL:
Cheesadilla
› **536** calories
› **34** g fat
(**19** g saturated)
› **1,174** mg sodium

WEIGHT LOSS

Salads always seem like the best choice, but what goes in and on top of the salad says it all. If you choose the California Grilled Chicken salad and lose the Asian Chicken Salad once a week at Jack Astor's, you will lose 9 lb (4 kg) in a year!

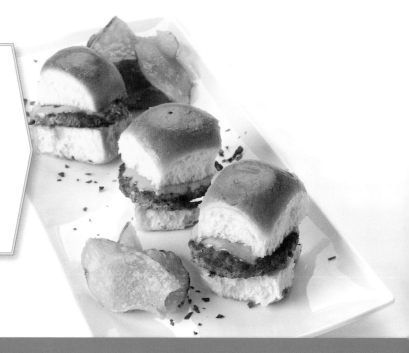

CHOOSE IT

CHEESEBURGER SLIDERS
(including secret sauce)

890 CALORIES
52 G FAT
1,640 MG SODIUM

JOEY

Joey has over 19 locations through-out British Columbia, Alberta, Man-itoba, Ontario and Washington State. Executive chef Chris Mills is the VP of Culinary and is renowned for taking classic dishes and put-ting a global spin on them. Joey is known for its upscale bar, res-taurant and sports bar, along with its attractive servers and host-esses, all dressed in black cocktail attire. The menu offers appetizers, sandwiches, Asian-inspired Wok 'n' Sauté, seafood, steaks, chicken, ribs, desserts and a number of sides. Nutritional information is clearly displayed online.

Why choose it? If you want to avoid overeating at Joey, the slid-ers are a better choice than the Earth and Surf Calamari because the beef and cheese in the sliders will fill you up faster. This option also has half the calories and 20 g less fat than the calamari dish.

ALSO CHOOSE

SANDWICH:
Hi-Rise Bacon Cheddar Burger
(including fries)
› **1,800** calories
› **105** g fat
› **2,820** mg sodium
› **155** g carbohydrates

MEAT DINNER ENTRÉE:
Steak and King Crab
(7 oz/198 g, including coleslaw)
› **1,180** calories
› **77** g fat
› **4,260** mg sodium
› **14** g carbohydrates

WOK 'N' SAUTÉ:
Panang Prawn Curry Bowl
› **680** calories
› **21** g fat
› **840** mg sodium

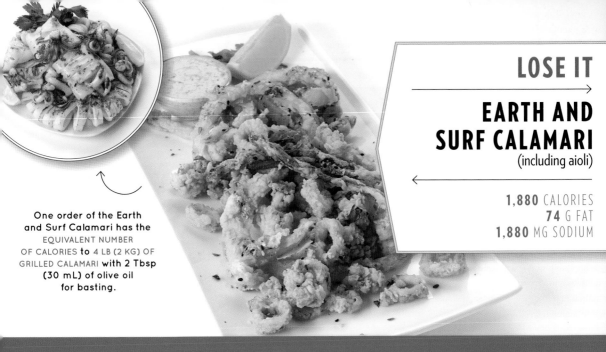

One order of the Earth and Surf Calamari has the **EQUIVALENT NUMBER OF CALORIES to** 4 LB (2 KG) OF GRILLED CALAMARI **with** 2 Tbsp (30 mL) of olive oil for basting.

LOSE IT

EARTH AND SURF CALAMARI
(including aioli)

1,880 CALORIES
74 G FAT
1,880 MG SODIUM

JOEY

Why lose it? This calamari, although made with seafood and vegetable, is battered and deep-fried. Now add an oil-based aioli on the side, and you'll understand why you have over a day's worth of calories, fat and sodium!

EXERCISE

Earth and Surf is an appropriate name for this deep-fried calamari and vegetable dish, since you will need to run for an hour and then swim for an hour to burn off the 1,880 calories and 74 g of fat.

ALSO LOSE

SANDWICH:
Beef Dip
(including fries)
› **2,600** calories
› **148** g fat
› **4,200** mg sodium
› **263** g carbohydrates

MEAT DINNER ENTRÉE:
Baby Back BBQ Ribs
(including barbeque sauce, rice)
› **2,380** calories
› **116** g fat
› **2,130** mg sodium
› **234** g carbohydrates

WOK 'N' SAUTÉ:
Bombay Butter Chicken
(including rice, grilled naan)
› **1,295** calories
› **76** g fat
› **830** mg sodium

→

SUMMER STRAWBERRY
(14 oz)

←

140 CALORIES
0 G FAT
35 G SUGAR

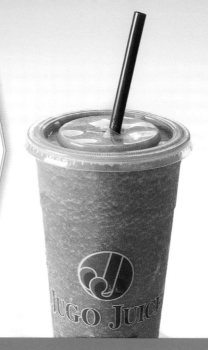

JUGO JUICE

Jugo Juice was founded in Calgary in 1998 with the goal of offering healthy alternatives to mainstream fast-food fare. Owners Derek Brock and Jason Cunningham are both former Starbucks baristas and hope to be catalysts for change in the food and beverage industry. With smoothies—billed as "the medicine chest of the future"—as its signature product, Jugo Juice now has over 100 locations across Canada. The smoothies contain over five servings of fruit in each 24 oz (680 g) cup. Nutritional information is provided online.

Why choose it? The Summer Strawberry smoothie is the reason you go to a Jugo Juice to start with. It has a variety of natural fruits combined into one drink—with half the calories, sugar and carbs of the Banana Buzz, plus no fat!

→

ALSO CHOOSE

TROPICAL SMOOTHIE:
Pineapple Powerzone
> **246** calories
> **0.2** g fat
> **62** g carbohydrates
> **53** g sugar

JUICE:
Carrot Juice
(14 oz/397 g)
> **123** calories
> **0** g fat
> **26** g carbohydrates
> **23** g sugar

JUICE:
Max Veg Juice
(14 oz/397 g)
> **83** calories
> **0** g fat
> **17** g carbohydrates
> **14** g sugar

↓

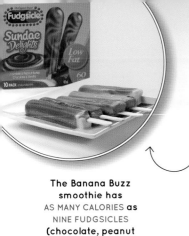

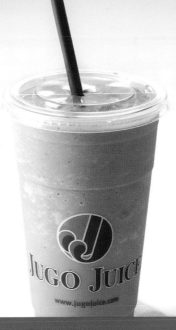

The Banana Buzz smoothie has AS MANY CALORIES as NINE FUDGSICLES (chocolate, peanut butter and vanilla).

LOSE IT

BANANA BUZZ
(14 oz)

302 CALORIES
5 G FAT
48 G SUGAR

JUGO JUICE

Why lose it? They don't call it "Buzz" for nothing. It has as much caffeine as a cup of coffee. The frozen yogurt, even though it's low fat, ups the calories and fat content—and it has over two days' worth of sugar!

ALSO LOSE

TROPICAL SMOOTHIE:
Coppa Banana
› **322** calories
› **0.4** g fat
› **81** g carbohydrates
› **69** g sugar

JUICE:
Apple Juice
(14 oz/397 g)
› **210** calories
› **0** g fat
› **53** g carbohydrates
› **45** g sugar

JUICE:
Orange Juice
(14 oz/397 g)
› **195** calories
› **0** g fat
› **45** g carbohydrates
› **37** g sugar

HOME COOKING

Avoid smoothies that contain frozen yogurt or ice cream. You don't need the extra calories and fat. Nor do you need the 24 oz (680 g) size, which equals 3 cups (750 mL). To make a great fruit smoothie at home, blend half a cup (125 mL) of lower-fat milk, half a cup of lower-fat fruit yogurt, one small banana and half a cup of orange juice. This serves four and contains only 100 calories and 1 g of fat!

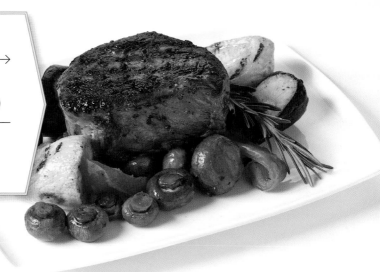

→

SIRLOIN STEAK
(12 oz/340 g, including vegetables)

←

511 CALORIES
22 G FAT (**8** G SATURATED)
651 MG SODIUM

PART 1 THE KEG

The Keg Steakhouse, originally The Keg and Cleaver, was founded in 1971 in North Vancouver by George Tidball. It now operates in all provinces except Prince Edward Island. There are also locations in Arizona, Texas, Washington State and Colorado. The Keg is well known for buying up historical manors and turning them into restaurants. The menu features steaks, prime rib, shellfish, salads and desserts, as well as its escargot and Mushrooms Neptune (mushroom caps stuffed with shrimp, crab, cream cheese, garlic

continued on page 74

Why choose it? This sirloin steak is larger than the prime rib cut and still has fewer calories and 30 percent less fat. The vegetables have only 55 calories compared with the 300-calorie mushrooms that come with the prime rib.

→

ALSO CHOOSE

APPETIZER:
Scallops & Bacon
(including cocktail sauce)
› **260** calories
› **15** g fat
   (**5** g saturated)
› **744** mg sodium

CHICKEN:
Teriyaki Chicken
(including dipping sauce)
› **455** calories
› **9** g fat
   (**2** g saturated)
› **831** mg sodium

CHILDREN'S MEAL:
Sirloin Steak
(not including sides)
› **244** calories
› **11** g fat
   (**4** g saturated)
› **559** mg sodium
› **0** g carbohydrates

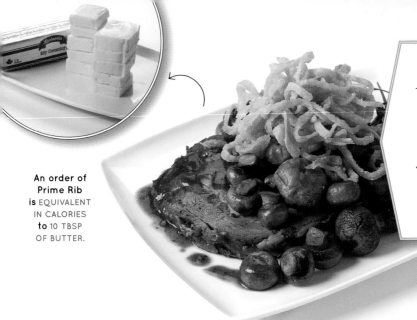

LOSE IT

PRIME RIB
(10 oz/283 g, including mushrooms,
jus, horseradish, frizzled onions)

1,050 CALORIES
59 G FAT (**16** G SATURATED)
2,543 MG SODIUM

THE KEG PART 1

Why lose it? Prime rib contains 35 to 45 percent fat, the highest of all other cuts. The fat is marbled, so it's not easy to trim away, and the jus from the meat also contains the fat from the beef. Add cremini mushrooms sautéed with excess fat and frizzled onions and you have three-quarters of a day's worth of calories, one day's worth of fat and over a day's worth of sodium!

NUTRITION

Beef cuts vary considerably in terms of fat and calories. An 8 oz (227 g) serving of flank steak has 540 calories and 11 g of fat, strip loin has 480 calories and 21 g of fat, rib-eye has 575 calories and 30 g of fat, T-bone has 575 calories and 27 g of fat, tenderloin has 471 calories and 19 g of fat and top sirloin has 420 calories and 15 g of fat.

ALSO LOSE

APPETIZER:
Tempura Snap Peas & Asparagus
(including soy dipping sauce)
› **641** calories
› **45** g fat
  (**4** g saturated)
› **412** mg sodium

CHICKEN:
Chicken Oscar
› **884** calories
› **60** g fat
  (**7** g saturated)
› **982** mg sodium

CHILDREN'S MEAL:
Mini Burgers
(not including sides)
› **364** calories
› **23** g fat
  (**10** g saturated)
› **624** mg sodium
› **26** g carbohydrates

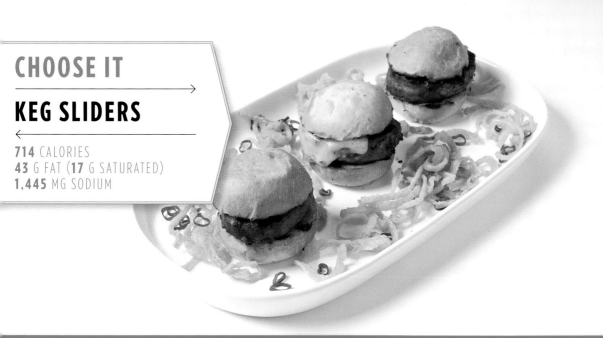

PART 2 THE KEG

continued from page 72

and herbs). The Keg aims to offer "quality, comfort and value." The website has a health guide with tips on how to make better choices and a diabetes guide, allergy guide and nutritional charts.

Why choose it? Even with ground prime rib, Swiss cheese, barbecue and blue cheese sauces, you're still getting fewer calories and less fat of the Chicken Wings.

ALSO CHOOSE

SALADS:

Keg Caesar
› **289** calories
› **20** g fat
   (**4** g saturated)
› **776** mg sodium

SIDE:

Roasted Garlic Mashed Potatoes
› **379** calories
› **23** g fat
   (**11** g saturated)
› **826** mg sodium

DESSERT:

Billy Miner Pie
› **573** calories
› **31** g fat
   (**15** g saturated)

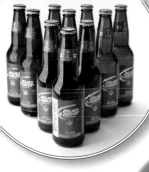

One order of
Chicken Wings has
AS MANY CALORIES
as TEN 12 fl oz
(370 mL) BUDWEISER
LAGERS (4.2 percent
alcohol).

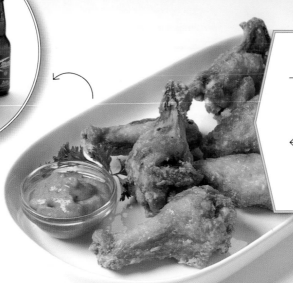

→

LOSE IT

CHICKEN WINGS
(including hot sauce)

←

1,100 CALORIES
82 G FAT (**23** G SATURATED)
1,237 MG SODIUM

THE KEG PART 2

Why lose it? Chicken wings have a high fat content because of the skin and little actual meat. To add insult to injury, these crispy (deep-fried) wings have about three-quarters of a day's worth of calories and sodium and over a day's worth of fat and saturated fat.

ALSO LOSE

SALADS:
Iceberg Wedge
(inclues bacon bits, blue cheese, blue cheese dressing)
› **474** calories
› **42** g fat
  (**13** g saturated)
› **989** mg sodium

SIDE:
Onion Rings
(including chipotle ranch sauce)
› **587** calories
› **22** g fat
  (**3** g saturated)
› **2,785** mg sodium

DESSERT:
Crème Brûlée
› **855** calories
› **61** g fat
  (**39** g saturated)

TRIVIA

If you enjoy eating at the Keg a couple of times a week, choose the Keg Sliders and lose the crispy Chicken Wings—you'll lose 12 lb (5 kg) in a year! The sliders have cheese, blue cheese sauce and barbecue sauce, so you're hardly depriving yourself!

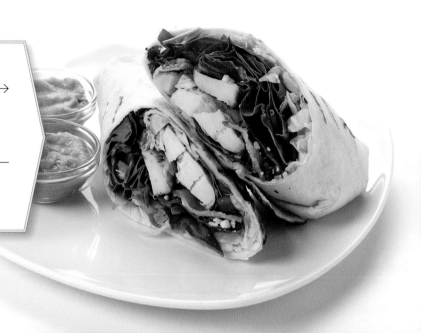

CALIFORNIA CHICKEN WRAP

←

660 CALORIES
32 G FAT (**12** G SATURATED)
1,660 MG SODIUM

KELSEY'S

Kelsey's Restaurant is a division of Cara Operations Ltd. with locations in Ontario, Manitoba, British Columbia and Alberta. The company mandate is to ensure that customers feel comfortable and at home. The menu includes appetizers, salads, pastas, entrées, sandwiches, burgers and kids' items, all at affordable prices. Nutritional information can be downloaded from the menu section of the website, and allergy information is also available. Healthier options are not highlighted, so check the nutrients in each item you might want to order.

Why choose it? This item has 400 fewer calories, 15 g less fat and half the sodium of the Pulled Pork Sandwich. It's delicious with hummus, guacamole, bacon and feta.

ALSO CHOOSE

PASTA AND FLATBREADS:
Balsamic Chicken Rigatoni
› **860** calories
› **36** g fat
 (**12** g saturated)
› **1,270** mg sodium

SIDES:
Yukon Gold Mashed Potatoes
› **200** calories
› **8** g fat
 (**4** g saturated)

CHILDREN'S MEAL:
Cheesy Alfredo Penne
› **300** calories
› **11** g fat
 (**5** g saturated)

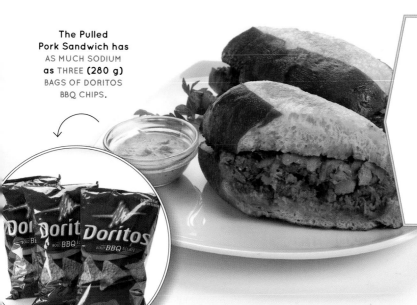

The Pulled Pork Sandwich has AS MUCH SODIUM as THREE **(280 g)** BAGS OF DORITOS BBQ CHIPS.

LOSE IT

→

PULLED PORK SANDWICH

(including Guinness barbecue sauce)

←

1,060 CALORIES
47 G FAT (**16** G SATURATED)
3,300 MG SODIUM

KELSEY'S

Why lose it? Pulled pork comes from the pork shoulder or butt, and the fatty and highly caloric parts of the pig. The pork is then mixed with some of the fat it was roasted in. Add cheeses and a pretzel bun, and you'll understand why you have about three-quarters of your daily calories, almost all your daily fat and 2.5 days' sodium!

ALSO LOSE

PASTA AND FLATBREADS:
BBQ Chicken Flatbread
› **1,250** calories
› **53** g fat (**25** g saturated)
› **4,040** mg sodium

SIDES:
Skillet of Mushrooms
› **330** calories
› **32** g fat (**6** g saturated)

CHILDREN'S MEAL:
Mini Cheeseburger
› **460** calories
› **27** g fat (**12** g saturated)

TRIVIA

Pulled pork is a form of barbequed pork where the meat is cooked on a low heat and becomes so tender that it can actually be "pulled" or easily torn into small, stringy pieces. Its popularity was once confined to the Southern United States, but its appeal has spread internationally in recent years.

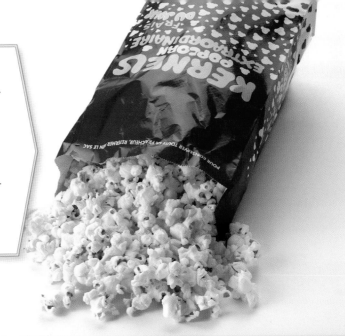

CHOOSE IT

→

BUTTERSALT POPCORN
(small, 9-cup/2 L bag)

409 CALORIES
21 G FAT (**2** G SATURATED)
352 MG SODIUM

KERNELS

Kernels was established in 1983 and is now the largest popcorn retailer in the world, with 70 stores across Canada and two more locations in South Korea and California. Its mission is to change plain old popcorn forever by adding a variety of savoury, sweet and spicy flavours and seasonings, some decadent and some low fat. Kernels' popcorn is air popped or popped in sunflower oil and has no trans fats. Dry seasonings add to the flavours but watch out for the sodium content. Detailed nutritionals are on the website.

Why choose it? The name is deceiving; "buttersalt" refers to the seasoning flavour rather than the addition of real butter. Therefore it's healthier than the Double-Butter popcorn.

ALSO CHOOSE

CARAMEL POPCORN:
Air Caramel
› **756** calories
› **16** g fat
   (**9** g saturated)
› **72** g sugar

CHEESE VS. CARAMEL:
Say Cheese
› **540** calories
› **32** g fat
› **1,100** mg sodium

SEASONING:
Onion Ranch
(2 tsp/10 mL)
› **20** calories
› **0** g fat
› **320** mg sodium

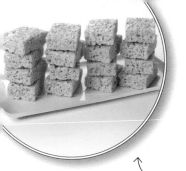

A small bag of Double-Butter Popcorn has AS MUCH FAT as 16 pre-packaged 22 g RICE KRISPIE TREATS.

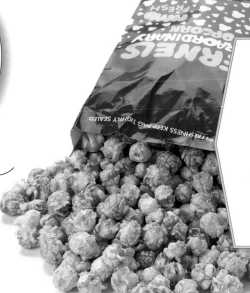

DOUBLE-BUTTER POPCORN
(small, 9-cup/2 L bag)

1,380 CALORIES
42 G FAT (**24** G SATURATED)
1,800 MG SODIUM

KERNELS

Why lose it? In this case, the name spells it out! A small bag of Double Butter can go pretty fast when you're mindlessly snacking! The first three ingredients in this flavour are sugar, butter and glucose, and that translates into calories and fat. You've got three-quarters of your day's worth of calories, sodium and total fat and your entire day's worth of saturated fat.

ALSO LOSE

CARAMEL POPCORN:
Creamy Caramel
› **1,320** calories
› **42** g fat
  (**24** g saturated)
› **114** g sugar

CHEESE VS. CARAMEL:
Low-Fat Caramel
› **900** calories
› **11** g fat
› **1,350** mg sodium

SEASONING:
White Cheddar
(2 tsp/10 mL)
› **30** calories
› **2** g fat
› **440** mg sodium

HOME COOKING

To make healthy popcorn at home, try using an air popper, which doesn't require any oil. Then have some fun: spray the popcorn with vegetable oil and sprinkle with your favourite dry seasonings or finely grated Parmesan cheese. You can also make popcorn in your microwave by taking a handful of kernels, placing them in a paper bag, folding over the opening and microwaving on high for about two minutes, or until you no longer hear the popping. Then add vegetable spray and seasoning.

CHOOSE IT

ORIGINAL RECIPE BREAST
(2 pieces)

320 CALORIES
12 G FAT (**2** G SATURATED)
880 MG SODIUM

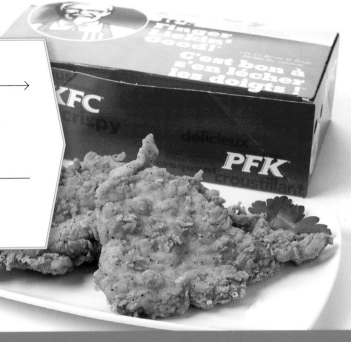

KFC

KFC (Kentucky Fried Chicken) was founded and based in Louisville, Kentucky, by Colonel Harland Sanders in 1952. It now has over 20,000 restaurants in 110 countries, most recently Kenya. Its famous secret Original Recipe is fried chicken with 11 herbs and spices. The chicken is grain fed. KFC has expanded its original menu and now offers chicken that is lower in calories, fat and sodium.

Why choose it? The fried breaded white meat saves on calories and fat compared with the dark meat. Three ounces of raw white chicken meat has only 168 calories and 5 g of fat versus dark meat, which has 320 calories and 12 g of fat.

ALSO CHOOSE

CHICKEN:
Crispy Chicken Strips
(3 pieces, 165 g)
› **330** calories
› **15** g fat
  (**1** g saturated)
› **1,200** mg sodium

BOWLS:
Chicken Bowl
(large, 16 oz/454 g)
› **560** calories
› **23** g fat
  (**4** g saturated)
› **1,520** mg sodium

SIDE:
Mashed Potatoes
(medium, 9 oz/268 g)
› **180** calories
› **0** g fat
› **2** g sugar
› **660** mg sodium

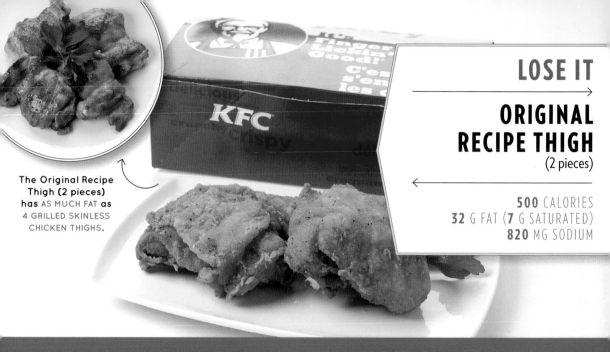

LOSE IT

ORIGINAL RECIPE THIGH
(2 pieces)

500 CALORIES
32 G FAT (**7** G SATURATED)
820 MG SODIUM

KFC

Why lose it? KFC's Original Recipe Chicken is always battered and deep-fried, which spells mega calories and fat. But two pieces of dark thigh meat has 180 more calories and 20 g more fat than the two pieces of white chicken.

ALSO LOSE

CHICKEN:
Popcorn Chicken
(small, 5 oz/142 g)
› **525** calories
› **34** g fat
  (**3** g saturated)
› **1,290** mg sodium

BOWLS:
Poutine
› **860** calories
› **48** g fat
  (**12** g saturated)
› **2,450** mg sodium

SIDE:
Corn
(medium)
› **290** calories
› **3** g fat
› **13** g sugar
› **0** mg sodium

TRIVIA

The recipe for KFC's fried chicken coating is so secret that to this day it's locked away in a high-security vault in Louisville, Kentucky, and very few people know the Colonel's secret blend. Even mixing the recipe is a high-security event. There are different KFC teams in different buildings and departments who mix parts of the recipe before it's all combined and mixed in a top-secret location! Who would have thought?

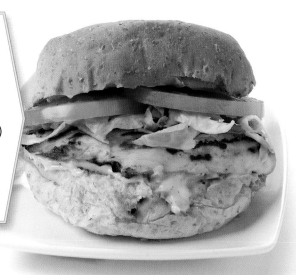

CHICK'N LICK'N BURGER
(including Guk sauce, whole wheat bun)

291 CALORIES
8 G FAT (**1** G SATURATED)
974 MG SODIUM

LICK'S

Lick's was launched in 1980 and now has over 24 locations in Ontario. It started with a huge hamburger patty grilled over charcoal and served with a special mayo-and-garlic sauce called Guk. Using lean, ground, pasteurized Canadian beef for their classic beef burgers, Lick's also offers vegan soy chicken and turkey burgers. When looking up nutritional information online, be sure to account for buns and toppings, as most are not included.

Why choose it? This grilled chicken burger is served on a whole wheat bun, which has fewer calories and less sodium than a regular hamburger bun. So feel free to add the special mayo-based "Guk" sauce. Load your burger up with veggies, and you've got close to half the calories and a third of the fat as the Nature Burger.

ALSO CHOOSE

OTHER MEAL 1:
Chili
(including whole wheat bun)
› **279** calories
› **8** g fat
   (**3** g saturated fat)
› **705** mg sodium

OTHER MEAL 2:
Veggie Chili
› **250** calories
› **8** g fat
   (**3** g saturated)
› **1,050** mg sodium

CHILDREN'S MEAL:
Kid's Nature Burger
› **296** calories
› **8** g fat
   (**8** g saturated fat)
› **557** mg sodium

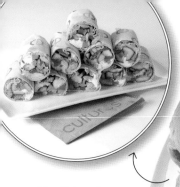

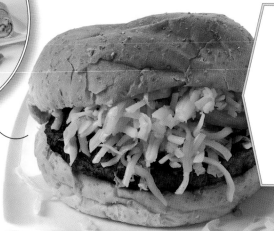

The Nature Burger has AS MUCH FAT as FIVE GRILLED VEGETABLE WRAPS from Cultures Restaurant.

NATURE BURGER
(including cheese, hamburger bun)

576 CALORIES
21 G FAT (**10** G SATURATED)
1,184 MG SODIUM

LICK'S

Why lose it? We tend to think that a veggie burger has to be the healthiest choice. But this burger lists hydrogenated vegetable oil as its third ingredient. That's the bad kind of fat! The regular hamburger bun alone has 268 calories and 450 mg of sodium!

ALSO LOSE

OTHER MEAL 1:
BLT
› **561** calories
› **25** g fat
  (**4** g saturated)
› **1,480** mg sodium

OTHER MEAL 2:
Caesar Salad
(regular size)
› **500** calories
› **30** g fat
  (**8** g saturated)
› **1,700** mg sodium

CHILDREN'S MEAL:
Nature Wrap
› **380** calories
› **15** g fat
  (**5** g saturated)
› **1,090** mg sodium

EXERCISE

After consuming your Nature Burger, you'd better go for a two-hour nature walk to burn off those 576 calories! Or shave off 268 calories and 450 mg of sodium by ordering the whole wheat bun rather than the regular hamburger bun. Then you'll only need to walk an hour!

CHOOSE IT

BLACK PEPPER CHICKEN

160 CALORIES
10 G FAT (**1.5** G SATURATED)
4 G SUGAR
640 MG SODIUM

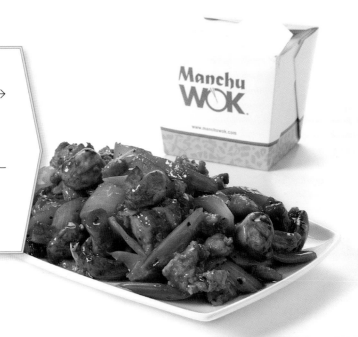

MANCHU WOK

Manchu Wok was founded in 1980 in Peterborough, and has since expanded nationally as well as internationally into the U.S., Japan and Korea. It is now owned by Hong Kong's largest Chinese fast-food chain, Coral Holdings Limited. With over 200 locations, Manchu Wok offers North America's version of Chinese cuisine with no MSG. Nutritional info is online; items that are trans-fat free, low in cholesterol or saturated fat and spicy are highlighted. Most items on the menu are under 450 calories with less than 20 g of fat.

Why choose it? The chicken is stir-fried rather than deep-fried, and the sauce is savoury instead of sweet. With almost 300 fewer calories than the Honey Garlic Chicken, and less than half the fat, this is definitely the better choice.

ALSO CHOOSE

BEEF:
Beef & Broccoli
› **190** calories
› **12** g fat
  (**1** g saturated)
› **700** mg sodium

PORK:
BBQ Pork
› **250** calories
› **11** g fat
  (**2** g saturated)
› **730** mg sodium
› **13** g sugar

NOODLES:
Lo Mein Noodles
› **350** calories
› **17** g fat
  (**1** g saturated)
› **870** mg sodium

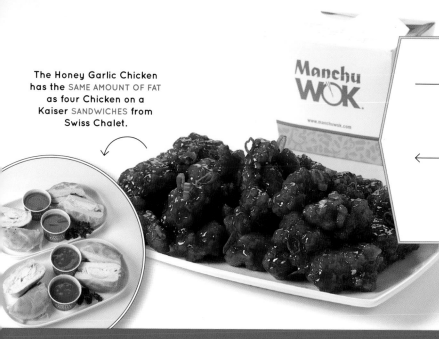

The Honey Garlic Chicken **has the** SAME AMOUNT OF FAT **as four Chicken on a Kaiser** SANDWICHES **from Swiss Chalet.**

LOSE IT

HONEY GARLIC CHICKEN

450 CALORIES
22 G FAT (**3** G SATURATED)
31 G SUGAR
890 MG SODIUM

MANCHU WOK

Why lose it? Even though the chicken is described as "lightly battered," it's still drenched in oil while deep-fried. Add the sweet honey sauce and you'll understand the high calories, fat and sugar.

ALSO LOSE

BEEF:
Ginger Beef
> **350** calories
> **22** g fat
  (**3** g saturated)
> **670** mg sodium

PORK:
Sweet & Sour Pork
> **350** calories
> **20** g fat
  (**2** g saturated)
> **540** mg sodium
> **19** g sugar

NOODLES:
Shanghai Noodles
> **410** calories
> **14** g fat
  (**1** g saturated)
> **1,620** mg sodium

HOME COOKING

A wok is a basic and versatile vessel used in Chinese cooking. You can use it to steam, stir-fry, braise, boil and deep-fry (not what I recommend). Food cut into small chunks is cooked quickly, easily and evenly in a small amount of oil. Your wok should never be more than one-third to one-half full when you are cooking to ensure food is heated throughout. When buying a wok, either purchase one made from carbon steel or cast iron, which has better heat retention than Teflon-coated ones or those made from aluminum.

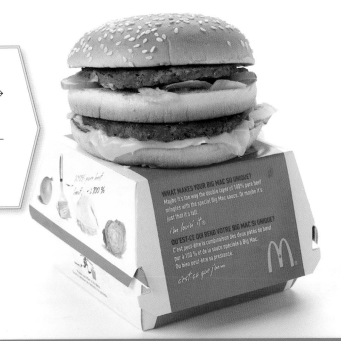

→

CHOOSE IT

BIG MAC

540 CALORIES
29 G FAT (**10** G SATURATED)
1,020 MG SODIUM

PART 1 McDONALD'S

McDonald's is known as the world's largest fast-food restaurant chain. The first Canadian McDonald's opened in 1967 in Richmond, BC. The chain had expanded nationally by the late '70s, and today there are over 1,400 restaurants across Canada, employing over 77,000 people. McDonald's is one of the largest employers of Canadian youth and is also known for its charitable activities benefiting children.

McDonald's has reinvented itself many times to keep up with its patrons' changing tastes while still

continued on page 88

Why choose it? Even two regular patties don't come close to the fat and calories of the Angus Burger. You're saving 240 calories and 18 g of fat. The Big Mac sauce adds an extra 100 calories and 10 g of fat, so try going without it!

ALSO CHOOSE

BREAKFAST SANDWICH:
Egg McMuffin
> **290** calories
> **12** g fat
  (**4** g saturated)
> **760** mg sodium

SNACK:
Cheeseburger
> **300** calories
> **12** g fat
  (**6** g saturated)
> **750** mg sodium

DESSERT:
Smarties McFlurry
(large/449 g)
> **580** calories
> **17** g fat
  (**11** g saturated)
> **83** g sugar
> **240** mg sodium

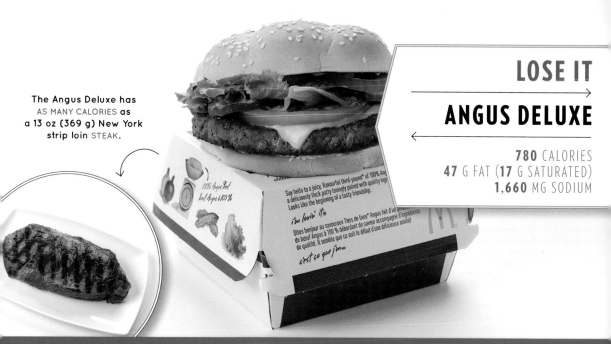

The Angus Deluxe has AS MANY CALORIES as a 13 oz (369 g) New York strip loin STEAK.

LOSE IT

ANGUS DELUXE

780 CALORIES
47 G FAT (**17** G SATURATED)
1,660 MG SODIUM

McDONALD'S PART 1

Why lose it? Angus beef is usually fattier beef. The patty alone is 320 calories and 23 g of fat. The premium (meaning bigger!) bun adds another 240 calories and 540 mg of sodium.

ALSO LOSE

BREAKFAST SANDWICH:
Bacon & Egg on Multigrain Bagel
› **620** calories
› **28** g fat
  (**8** g saturated)
› **1,090** mg sodium

SNACK:
McChicken Sandwich
› **470** calories
› **27** g fat
  (**5** g saturated)
› **790** mg sodium

DESSERT:
Triple-Thick Chocolate Banana Milkshake
(large/449 mg)
› **1,130** calories
› **29** g fat
  (**17** g saturated)
› **158** g sugar
› **820** mg sodium

TRIVIA

» McDonald's serves over 64 million customers daily in over 119 countries.
» Every day, 0.5 percent of the world's population visits McDonald's.
» McDonald's is the largest property owner in the world. It is also the largest toy distributor in the world.

CHOOSE IT

→

SPICY THAI SALAD
(including grilled chicken,
Thai sauce, vinaigrette)

←

330 CALORIES
12 G FAT (**1** G SATURATED)
920 MG SODIUM

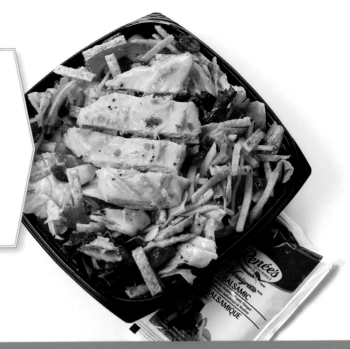

PART 2 McDONALD'S

continued from page 86

staying true to its original fast-food appeal.

After receiving bad press regarding the quality of its food, the company put detailed information on its website about all ingredients used. The website is very informative; it has a nutritional calculator with menu choices for those wanting healthier choices, items under 500 calories, diabetes-friendly items, healthier children's choices and foods with 20 g of fat or less.

Why choose it? The grilled chicken, vinaigrette dressing and small portion of whole wheat noodles make this a healthier—and tastier—choice.

→

ALSO CHOOSE

SNACK:
Chipotle Grilled Chicken Wrap
› **230** calories
› **6** g fat
   (**3** g saturated)
› **520** mg sodium

HAPPY MEAL:
Cheeseburger
(including apple slices, apple juice)
› **510** calories
› **13** g fat
   (**6** g saturated)
› **810** mg sodium

DESSERT:
Strawberry Sundae
› **290** calories
› **6** g fat
   (**4** g saturated)
› **130** mg sodium
› **44** g sugar

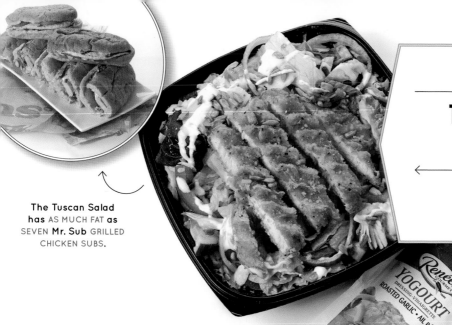

LOSE IT →

TUSCAN SALAD
(including crispy chicken,
yogurt dressing)

560 CALORIES
34 G FAT (**7** G SATURATED)
760 MG SODIUM

The Tuscan Salad
has AS MUCH FAT as
SEVEN **Mr. Sub** GRILLED
CHICKEN SUBS.

McDONALD'S PART 2

Why lose it? The chicken is deep-fried, and alone has double the calories and six times the fat of the grilled chicken. Renee's makes delicious dressings, but this option sounds healthier than it is. The dressing alone has 130 calories and 13 g of fat.

ALSO LOSE

SNACK:
Poutine
> **500** calories
> **27** g fat
   (**11** g saturated)
> **890** mg sodium

HAPPY MEAL:
Cheeseburger
(including mini fries, child-size chocolate banana triple-thick milkshake)
> **910** calories
> **30** g fat
   (**14** g saturated)
> **1,200** mg sodium

DESSERT:
Cinnamon Melts
> **460** calories
> **20** g fat
   (**8** g saturated)
> **400** mg sodium
> **19** g sugar

TRIVIA

» McDonald's use of red and yellow in its branding serves a purpose; those happen to be the colours that induce hunger.

» A new McDonald's opens somewhere in the world every six hours.

» Sweden has a ski-through McDonald's.

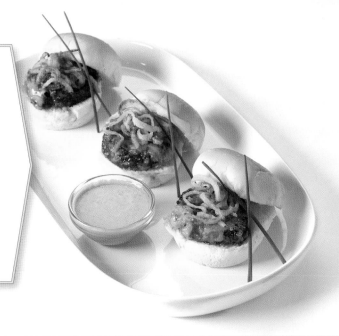

CHOOSE IT

→

KOBE-STYLE CLASSIC BEEF SLIDERS
(including sesame mustard sauce)

←

610 CALORIES
26 G FAT (**7** G SATURATED)
1,720 MG SODIUM

PART 1 MILESTONES

Milestones first opened in Vancouver in 1989 and became another Cara Operations chain with 38 locations across British Columbia, Alberta and Ontario. The restaurant is about inspired, familiar food with a twist. Milestones has a stylish and inviting atmosphere and likes to make its customers feel comfortable, serving up classic appetizers, share plates, signature salads, steaks and prime ribs, seafood, pasta bowls and burgers. There's a special Date Night menu for Wednesdays where two can dine

continued on page 92

Why choose it? Even though Kobe beef is the fattiest and most delicious of all cuts, these sliders with crispy onions strings are still a better choice of appetizer than the Hot Spinach and Artichoke Dip for calories and fat. The protein will fill you up more than the dip, so you might order a smaller entrée!

→

ALSO CHOOSE

ENTRÉE:
New York Striploin
(10 oz/283 g, including peppercorn sauce)
› **560** calories
› **23** g fat
  (**10** g saturated)
› **360** mg sodium

PASTA DISH:
Chicken Penne Asiago
(including cream sauce)
› **1,140** calories
› **60** g fat
  (**26** g saturated)
› **2,670** mg sodium

SANDWICH:
Chicken Burger
› **430** calories
› **14** g fat
  (**2** g saturated)
› **1,010** mg sodium

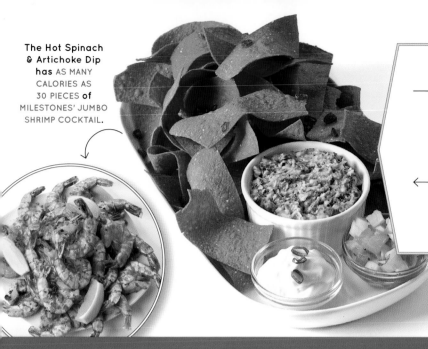

The Hot Spinach & Artichoke Dip has AS MANY CALORIES AS 30 PIECES of MILESTONES' JUMBO SHRIMP COCKTAIL.

HOT SPINACH & ARTICHOKE DIP
(including sour cream, salsa)

1,000 CALORIES
64 G FAT (**24** G SATURATED)
1,580 MG SODIUM

MILESTONES PART 1

Why lose it? Hot spinach and artichoke. What could be healthier? Think again! The cheeses, sour cream and massive amount of deep-fried tortilla chips on the side accounts for a large portion of your recommended daily calories, fat and saturated fat. Even sharing is not such a great idea!

ALSO LOSE

ENTRÉE:
Slow-Roasted AAA Prime Rib
(10 oz/283 g, including jus)
› **1,250** calories
› **103** g fat
  (**43** g saturated)
› **3,780** mg sodium

PASTA DISH:
Grilled Chicken Pesto Fettuccini
(including pesto cream sauce)
› **1,460** calories
› **94** g fat
  (**35** g saturated)
› **3,290** mg sodium

SANDWICH:
Spicy Thai Chicken Roll-Ups
(including aioli)
› **1,050** calories
› **48** g fat
  (**7** g saturated)
› **2,790** mg sodium

FOOD FACT

Kobe beef refers to cuts of beef from Wagyu cattle. Flavourful, tender and marbled with fat, this meat is considered the caviar of beef. It also has more calories and fat than traditional beef. Kobe beef is also eaten rolled up as "sushi" in Japan. To make the meat so tender, farmers isolate the cattle, add beer or sake to their food and massage the animals' backsides!

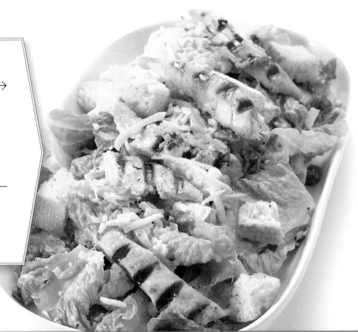

CHOOSE IT

GRILLED CHICKEN CAESAR SALAD
(including two cheeses, garlic, croutons, dressing)

620 CALORIES
45 G FAT (**8** G SATURATED)
1,340 MG SODIUM

continued from page 90

for $50 and a Girls' Night Out menu for Mondays, that features an appetizer and drink for $10. As a healthy initiative, Milestones includes a Gluten-Free-Favourites section on their menu as well as a section with items under 800 mg of sodium. Nutritionals are easily found online.

Why choose it? I rarely recommend a caesar salad, but this one is slightly smaller than most, with almost half the calories and fat of the Grilled Chicken Salad. You're still getting croutons, ciabatta and Reggiano cheese.

ALSO CHOOSE

BURGER VS. SANDWICH:
Milestone's Beef Burger
› **690** calories
› **30** g fat
   (**7** g saturated)
› **1,330** mg sodium

CHICKEN ENTRÉE:
Grilled Mediterranean Chicken
(including cheese)
› **680** calories
› **31** g fat
   (**10** g saturated)
› **1,900** mg sodium

DESSERT:
Ginger Caramel Apple Crisp
› **800** calories
› **31** g fat
   (**14** g saturated)
› **89** g sugar

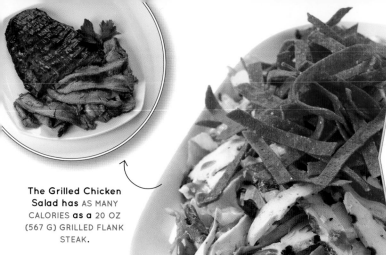

The Grilled Chicken Salad has AS MANY CALORIES as a 20 OZ (567 G) GRILLED FLANK STEAK.

LOSE IT

GRILLED CHICKEN SALAD

(including tortilla chips, vinaigrette, peanut sauce)

1040 CALORIES
82 G FAT (**8** G SATURATED)
1390 MG SODIUM

MILESTONES PART 2

Why lose it? Normally you'd think that a grilled chicken salad has to be better for you than a caesar, but not in this case. Read the fine print! The fried tortilla chips, peanut vinaigrette and peanut sauce give you a salad that has half your daily calories and a full day's worth of fat.

ALSO LOSE

BURGER VS. SANDWICH:
Prime Rib Beef Dip
(including gorgonzola butter)
› **1,070** calories
› **74** g fat
   (**28** g saturated)
› **1,280** mg sodium

CHICKEN ENTRÉE:
Portobello Mushroom Chicken
(including Regianno cream)
› **1,270** calories
› **71** g fat
   (**28** g saturated)
› **1,370** mg sodium

DESSERT:
The Cookie
(including vanilla gelato, caramel and chocolate sauces)
› **1,300** calories
› **69** g fat
   (**36** g saturated)
› **113** g sugar

TRIVIA

Traditional caesar salad dressings are a nutritional landmine. One tablespoon (15 mL) contains 90 calories and 10 g of fat. One caesar salad would easily have one-third of a cup (80 mL) of dressing, which means you are eating 540 calories and 60 g of fat just in the dressing! To lessen the fat, either buy reduced-fat caesar dressing or combine half the traditional with low-fat yogurt or low-fat sour cream. You'll reduce the calories and fat close to 50 percent.

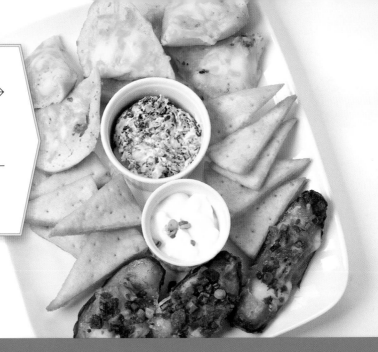

CHOOSE IT →

COOKHOUSE PLATTER

←

1,490 CALORIES
77 G FAT (**36** G SATURATED)
2,930 MG SODIUM

PART 1 MONTANA'S

Montana's, a subsidiary of Kelsey's, opened its doors in 1995 and now has over 85 locations across Canada. It specializes in anything grilled, smoked or saucy, including "fall off the bone" ribs, fresh Canadian AAA steak and slow-roasted barbecue rotisserie chicken. The restaurant has a casual, family atmosphere. Nutrition and allergy information is available online, but read carefully, as sides (such as sour cream, garlic bread, rice, seasonal vegetables, sauces and dips) are not included in the totals for main

continued on page 96

Why choose it? Assuming you'll be sharing this appetizer, which includes garlic bread, cheese, spinach dip and pita and potato skins with sour cream, you will save close to 1,000 calories, 60 g of fat, and 600 mg of sodium. Still, it's not the healthiest of choices!

ALSO CHOOSE

APPETIZER:	RIBS:	STEAK:
Hand-Dusted Calamari	**Ribs 'n' Chicken Combo**	**Cookhouse Top Sirloin**
(including Thai sauce)	(including barbecue sauce)	(12 oz/340 g)
› **470** calories	› **1,100** calories	› **500** calories
› **24** g fat (**2** g saturated)	› **70** g fat (**25** g saturated)	› **17** g fat (**7** g saturated)
› **460** mg sodium	› **1,000** mg sodium	› **690** mg sodium

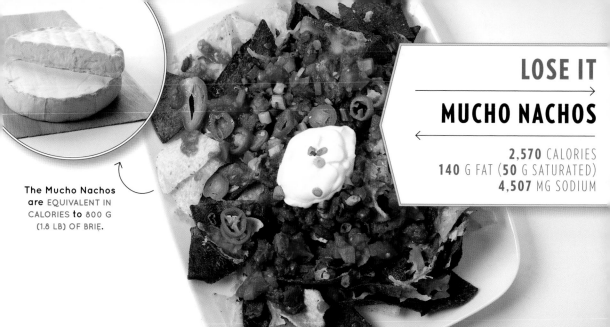

The Mucho Nachos **are** EQUIVALENT IN CALORIES **to** 800 G (1.8 LB) OF BRIE.

MUCHO NACHOS

2,570 CALORIES
140 G FAT (**50** G SATURATED)
4,507 MG SODIUM

MONTANA'S PART 1

Why lose it? Nachos are always a landmine of calories, fat, saturated fat, sodium and carbs, even if you're sharing. These over-the-top nutrients come from the deep-fried tortilla chips, beef chili, cheese and sour cream. This option is about one and a half days' worth of calories and two days' worth of fat, saturated fat and sodium.

HOME COOKING

Make your own tortilla chips that are baked, not deep-fried, but still delicious. Take any flavour of a large tortilla. Spray with vegetable oil, then sprinkle with seasonings of your choice, such as garlic or onion powder, Parmesan cheese, cayenne or paprika. Slice each tortilla into eight wedges and bake at 350ºF (175ºC) for 12 minutes, until lightly browned.

ALSO LOSE

APPETIZER:
Four Cheese Spinach Dip
(including fried pita chips)
› **1,160** calories
› **80** g fat
  (**27** g saturated)
› **1,630** mg sodium

RIBS:
Beef Ribs
(large, 540 g, including barbecue sauce)
› **1,800** calories
› **106** g fat
  (**45** g saturated)
› **1,780** mg sodium

STEAK:
Grilled Rib-Eye
(12 oz/340 g)
› **730** calories
› **53** g fat
  (**25** g saturated)
› **430** mg sodium

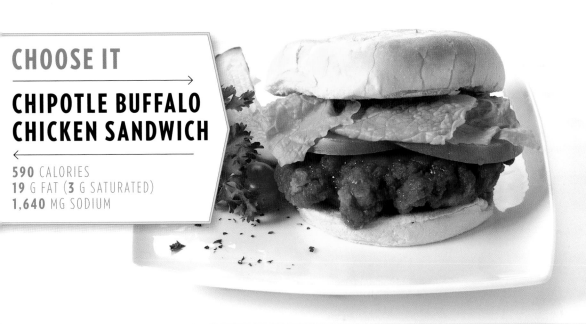

CHOOSE IT

CHIPOTLE BUFFALO CHICKEN SANDWICH

590 CALORIES
19 G FAT (**3** G SATURATED)
1,640 MG SODIUM

continued from page 94

dishes and must be calculated separately. Montana's doesn't offer a menu of "healthy choices" as of yet.

Why choose it? The chicken may be breaded, but the wing sauce doesn't compare in calories and fat to the caesar dressing in the Smokehouse Wrap. Coming in at under half the calories, sodium and fat, this is a far better choice.

ALSO CHOOSE

SIDE 1:
Garlic & Gravy Mashed Potatoes
› **110** calories
› **3** g fat
  (**1** g saturated)
› **2** g sugar
› **848** mg sodium

SIDE 2:
French Fries
› **400** calories
› **22** g fat
  (**2** g saturated)
› **1,060** mg sodium

CHILDREN'S MENU:
Pork Back Ribs
(including french fries, carrot sticks)
› **600** calories
› **31** g fat
  (**10** g saturated)
› **1,340** mg sodium

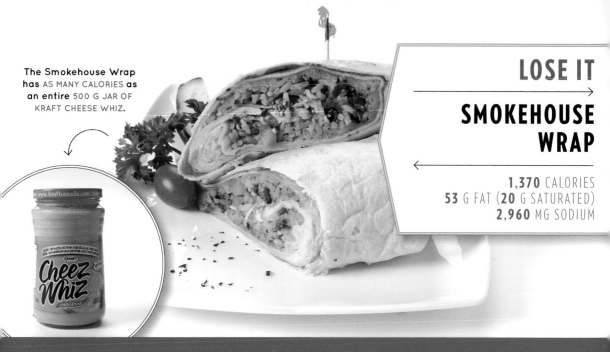

The Smokehouse Wrap has AS MANY CALORIES as an entire 500 G JAR OF KRAFT CHEESE WHIZ.

LOSE IT

SMOKEHOUSE WRAP

1,370 CALORIES
53 G FAT (**20** G SATURATED)
2,960 MG SODIUM

MONTANA'S PART 2

Why lose it? This wrap has pulled chicken rather than breaded. Pulled chicken is often combined with the fat it cooks in. Now add the bacon, cheese and caesar dressing, and you'll understand why you're getting almost three-quarters of your recommended daily calories, an entire day's worth of fat and saturated fat and close to two days' worth of sodium.

WEIGHT LOSS

If you choose the Chipotle Buffalo Chicken Sandwich and lose the Smokehouse Wrap once a week for a year, you will lose 12 lb (5 kg), without changing anything else about your lifestyle or eating habits!

ALSO LOSE

SIDE 1:
Skillet of Mushrooms
› **370** calories
› **32** g fat
  (**6** g saturated)
› **6** g sugar
› **270** mg sodium

SIDE 2:
Poutine
› **780** calories
› **49** g fat
  (**17** g saturated)
› **2,180** mg sodium

CHILDREN'S MEAL:
Jr. Beef Burger
(including caesar salad)
› **1,050** calories
› **70** g fat
  (**19** g saturated)
› **1,900** mg sodium

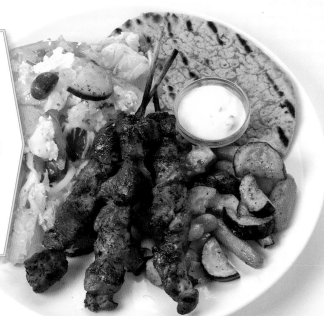

ORIGINAL PORK SOUVLAKI

(3 sticks, including tzatziki, pita, roasted vegetables, green salad)

1156 CALORIES
85 G FAT (**20** G SATURATED)
2,736 MG SODIUM

MR. GREEK

Mr. Greek first opened its doors in Greek Town, on the Danforth in Toronto, in 1988. Four years later, a second location opened in Scarborough. Today, there are 16 Mr. Greeks in the GTA, and the chain is considered one of the largest and fastest-growing Greek/Mediterranean restaurant franchises in North America. Mr. Greek is passionate about quality and gives its customers an enjoyable, relaxing environment. It also offers takeout and catering. Nutritional information has recently been released on the Mr. Greek website.

Why choose it? Pork is leaner than the lamb or beef, and the sides (roast vegetables and Greek salad) account for only about 300 calories. Still, this dish is three-quarters of your daily recommended calories, one and a half days' worth of fat and over a day's worth of sodium.

ALSO CHOOSE

CHICKEN:
Chicken Souvlaki
(including whole wheat pita, tzatziki)
› **537** calories
› **26** g fat
  (**3** g saturated)
› **756** mg sodium

SIDES:
Mr. Greek Potatoes
› **220** calories
› **6** g fat
  (**0** g saturated)
› **1,760** mg sodium

CHILDREN'S MEAL:
Super Hero Gyro
(3 oz/85 g beef and lamb, whole wheat pita)
› **205** calories
› **13** g fat
  (**1** g saturated)
› **267** mg sodium

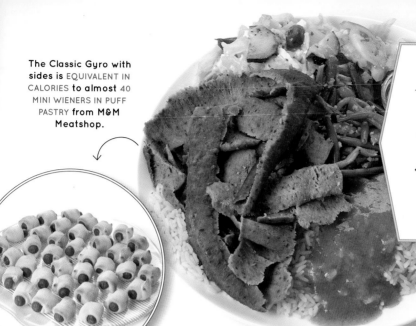

The Classic Gyro with sides is EQUIVALENT IN CALORIES **to almost** 40 MINI WIENERS IN PUFF PASTRY **from M&M Meatshop.**

LOSE IT

→

CLASSIC GYRO

(8 oz/227 g, including tzatziki, Greek salad, rice, sautéed green beans)

←

2,349 CALORIES
146 G FAT (**45** G SATURATED)
5,942 MG SODIUM

MR. GREEK

Why lose it? This meal contains almost a day's worth of calories and two days' worth of fat and saturated fat. Lamb and beef are higher in calories and fat than pork. But most shocking is that the sides of rice and green beans have 600 calories and 20 g of fat, and the dressing has 320 calories and 36 g of fat!

HEALTH FACT

Lamb is generally higher in calories and fat than beef, but the nutritional value is affected by the cut. One advantage is that lamb tends to have less marbling than beef. The leanest choices include loin, shank and leg, which are comparable to beef or pork in terms of calories and fat. A 3 oz (85 g) serving is about 160 calories, 8 g of fat and 3 g of saturated fat. However, some cuts of lamb, such as ground, can have 20 to 30 more calories per serving than their beef counterparts.

ALSO LOSE

CHICKEN:
Chicken Greek Wrap
(including Greek salad)
› **697** calories
› **32** g fat
  (**9** g saturated)
› **2,183** mg sodium

SIDES:
Mr. Greek Rice
› **786** calories
› **24** g fat
  (**5** g saturated)
› **2,535** mg sodium

CHILDREN'S MEAL:
Chicken Penne
› **813** calories
› **46** g fat
  (**16** g saturated)
› **301** mg sodium

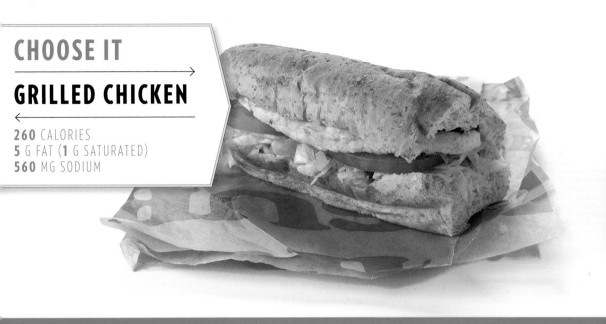

CHOOSE IT

GRILLED CHICKEN

260 CALORIES
5 G FAT (**1** G SATURATED)
560 MG SODIUM

MR. SUB

Mr. Sub, a Canadian chain founded in 1968, specializes in submarine sandwiches. It's come a long way since its first location in Toronto's hip Yorkville neighbourhood catered to patrons in bell-bottom jeans and tie-dyed shirts! With a mission to serve quality food and serve it fast, Mr. Sub was an immediate success and expanded quickly; it now has 335 locations across Canada. The website has an excellent nutritional table. All subs are under approximately 500 calories with no more than 20 g of fat. Sodium is an issue with some of the subs, mostly due to the deli meats used.

Why choose it? Grilled chicken is always low in calories, fat and sodium. The cheese and light mayo used here is lower in fat and calories than the buttermilk ranch sauce used in the Santa Fe Spicy Chicken.

ALSO CHOOSE

PANINI:
Classic Reuben
› **290** calories
› **7** g fat
  (**3** g saturated)
› **1,400** mg sodium

WRAP:
Smoked Turkey Breast
› **360** calories
› **9** g fat
  (**1** g saturated)
› **1,320** mg sodium

BREAKFAST SANDWICH:
Steak & Egg
› **355** calories
› **13** g fat
  (**5** g saturated)
› **892** mg sodium

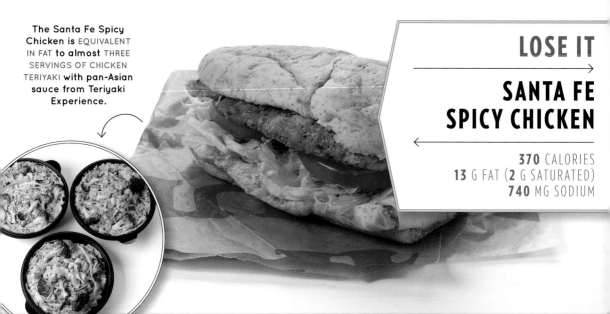

The Santa Fe Spicy Chicken is EQUIVALENT IN FAT to almost THREE SERVINGS OF CHICKEN TERIYAKI with pan-Asian sauce from Teriyaki Experience.

→←

LOSE IT

SANTA FE SPICY CHICKEN

370 CALORIES
13 G FAT (**2** G SATURATED)
740 MG SODIUM

MR. SUB

Why lose it? The name doesn't tell you the chicken is breaded and deep-fried. Buttermilk is a healthy, low-fat ingredient on its own, but the buttermilk ranch sauce adds oil or mayonnaise, which increases the calories and fat.

ALSO LOSE

PANINI:
Ultimate Cheddar Cheese Club
› **440** calories
› **18** g fat
  (**9** g saturated)
› **1,530** mg sodium

WRAP:
Albacore Tuna
› **460** calories
› **16** g fat
  (**1** g saturated)
› **1,100** mg sodium

BREAKFAST SANDWICH:
Sausage & Egg
› **505** calories
› **30** g fat
  (**10** g saturated)
› **1,200** mg sodium

FOOD FACT

The myth around buttermilk is that it is a buttery, high-fat milk. This couldn't be further from the truth. There is no butter in buttermilk, and it is lower in fat than whole milk. It has a yogurt-like flavour and is slightly thicker than regular milk. It is made by adding a lactic acid bacteria culture to skim milk, leaving it to ferment for 12 hours at a low temperature of 69ºF (21ºC). You can use buttermilk in recipes to replace low-fat yogurt or sour cream. To make your own buttermilk, just add 1 Tbsp (15 mL) of lemon juice or white vinegar to 1 cup (250 mL) of milk and let it sit for 10 minutes.

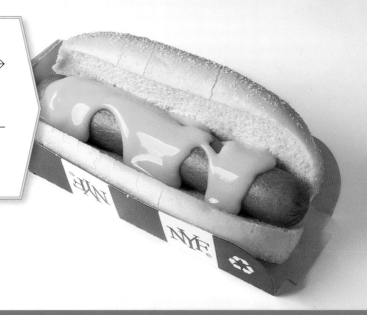

HOT DOG
(including cheese sauce)

←

435 CALORIES
21 G FAT (**7** G SATURATED)
1,270 MG SODIUM

NEW YORK FRIES

New York Fries is a privately owned Canadian franchise established in 1983. The founders, brothers Jason and Hal Gould, came up with the idea after eating some exceptionally good fries on a trip to New York. The New York Fries chain now has locations in Canada, Bahrain, Hong Kong, Macau and the United Arab Emirates. The fries are hand cut in the store throughout the day, with the skin left on. They are fried right when you order in non-hydrogenated sunflower oil. The result is a crisp, lightly golden french fry. The website has detailed nutritional information.

Why choose it? The hot dog at least gives you 17 g of protein, which will fill you up for longer than just the fries. Still, it's not the healthiest choice for a meal or snack, since it's made with processed meat.

→

ALSO CHOOSE

MEAL:
Works
(regular, 254 g)
› **880** calories
› **42** g fat
  (**6** g saturated)
› **1,110** mg sodium

SAUCE:
Gravy
(148 mL)
› **75** calories
› **2** g fat
  (**1** g saturated)
› **939** mg sodium

TOPPING:
Cheese Sauce
› **15** calories
› **0** g fat
  (**0** g saturated)
› **130** mg sodium

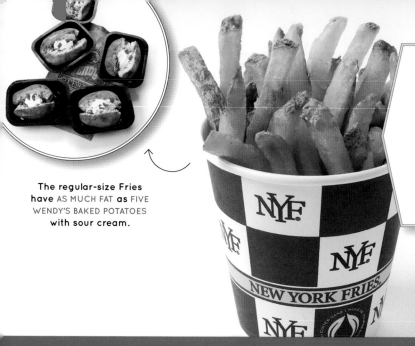

The regular-size Fries have AS MUCH FAT as FIVE WENDY'S BAKED POTATOES with sour cream.

NEW YORK FRIES

Why lose it? Fries are never a healthy choice, even when they have been hand cut with the skin left on and then cooked in non-hydrogenated sunflower oil! One order is one-third of your daily calories and half a day's worth of fat. Also, they are a higher glycemic food, raising your blood sugar quickly and leaving you hungry sooner. If you have to have fries, go for the small size.

HOME COOKING

Make your own potato wedges next time you crave fries. Preheat the oven to 375°F (190°C) and cut three large baking potatoes into eight wedges each. Place on a baking sheet sprayed with oil and sprinkle with olive oil, garlic powder, chili powder and grated Parmesan cheese. Bake for 20 minutes. Turn over, add the same seasonings and bake for another 20 minutes. Four wedges are 150 calories with 5 g of fat; the same size of restaurant fries typically has around 450 calories and 20 g of fat.

ALSO LOSE

MEAL:
Poutine
(regular, 320 g, including extra cheese curds)
› **1,120** calories
› **63** g fat
   (**21** g saturated)
› **1,640** mg sodium

SAUCE:
Sour Cream
(148 mL)
› **250** calories
› **24** g fat
   (**12** g saturated)
› **120** mg sodium

TOPPING:
Bacon
› **40** calories
› **3** g fat
   (**1** g saturated)
› **160** mg sodium

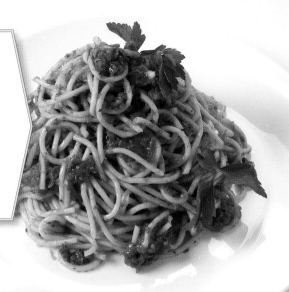

CHOOSE IT

→

SPAGHETTI WITH SPICY MEAT SAUCE

←

634 CALORIES
21 G FAT
652 MG SODIUM

THE OLD SPAGHETTI FACTORY

The Old Spaghetti Factory started in 1969 in Portland, Oregon, and has since grown to 40 locations internationally. Several of the restaurants are located in older warehouses and historic locations. The décor features antiques, chandeliers, brass headboards and footboards in the booths as well as a streetcar with seating inside.

The nutritionals are online, but they don't include the complimentary sides to the all-inclusive meal—salad, bread and ice cream—which add excess calories and fat.

Why choose it? You're always safer with this good old plain spaghetti without all the excess cheese, white sauce or eggs. With almost half the calories of the Lasagna with Meat Sauce and 40 percent less fat and sodium, you can afford the extras that come with the meal.

→

ALSO CHOOSE

APPETIZER:
Chicken Dippers
› **468** calories
› **10** g fat
› **927** mg sodium

SALAD:
Spinach Salad with Chicken
(including vinaigrette dressing)
› **428** calories
› **23** g fat
› **302** mg sodium

CHILDREN'S MEAL:
Spaghetti
(including meat sauce)
› **330** calories
› **7** g fat
› **385** mg sodium

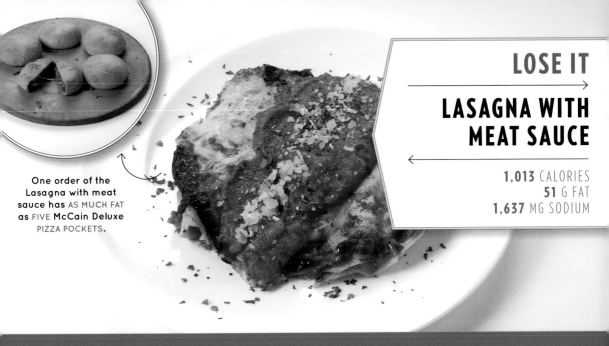

One order of the Lasagna with meat sauce has AS MUCH FAT as FIVE McCain Deluxe PIZZA POCKETS.

→

LOSE IT

LASAGNA WITH MEAT SAUCE

1,013 CALORIES
51 G FAT
1,637 MG SODIUM

THE OLD SPAGHETTI FACTORY

Why lose it? The minute you hear "Mama Pulosi's Secret Home-made Recipe," watch out. It's a secret for a reason. One dish, which includes three cheeses (Parmesan, mozzarella and ricotta) gives you three-quarters of your daily calories and almost a day's worth of fat and sodium. And remember, this doesn't include the complimentary bread, salad or ice cream!

EXERCISE

After you eat this traditional lasagna (with over 1,000 calories and 50 g of fat), get out and play soccer, Italy's national sport, for a couple of hours! That's what you'll need to burn off this dinner.

ALSO LOSE

APPETIZER:
Chicken Wings
(including spicy sauce)
› **770** calories
› **44** g fat
› **3,779** mg sodium

SALAD:
Mediterranean Salad
› **810** calories
› **60** g fat
› **811** mg sodium

CHILDREN'S MEAL:
Child Chicken & Fries
› **686** calories
› **15** g fat
› **1,878** mg sodium

PIÑA COLADA
(medium)

470 CALORIES
8 G FAT (**7** G SATURATED)
90 G SUGAR
100 MG SODIUM

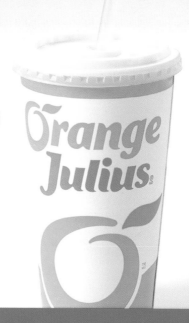

ORANGE JULIUS

Orange Julius dates back to the 1920s, opening in Los Angeles by Julius Freed. The Orange Julius was named the official drink at the New York World's Fair in 1964. In the 1980s, the chain introduced raw eggs as part of their blended drinks to add more protein, especially for body builders. Later on, the raw egg was replaced by bananas because of food safety concerns. Today, the Orange Julius menu consists of smoothies made with fruit, juice and frozen yogurt. There are also dairy-free options. Nutritionals are included online, but beware—the list is long and detailed.

Why choose it? Traditional piña coladas are filled with calories and saturated fat because they are made with coconut milk, but this version is much lighter. It also has half the calories, three times less fat and eight times less sodium than the Cool Mocha Julius, and you're consuming some real fruit! Nutritional information is based on medium-size (20 oz/567 g) drinks.

ALSO CHOOSE

PREMIUM FRUIT SMOOTHIES:
Mango Passion
› **290** calories
› **49** g sugar
› **67** g carbohydrates

JULIUS VS. COFFEE:
Raspberry Julius
› **350** calories
› **1** g fat
  (**0.3** g saturated)
› **89** g sugar

JULIUS JUICE:
Orange Julius
› **290** calories
› **0.5** g fat
  (**0.3** g saturated)
› **73** g sugar

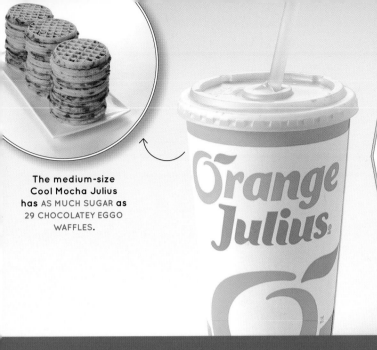

The medium-size
Cool Mocha Julius
has AS MUCH SUGAR as
29 CHOCOLATEY EGGO
WAFFLES.

LOSE IT

COOL MOCHA JULIUS
(medium)

820 CALORIES
16 G FAT (**13** G SATURATED)
127 G SUGAR
780 MG SODIUM

ORANGE JULIUS

Why lose it? You need a foreign translator to understand what's in this drink. But I can assume that the calories, fat and sugar come from the chocolate drink base. I'd shy away from drinking half your day's calorie and sodium intake, not to mention 32 tsp (480 mL), or three days' worth, of sugar! Nutritional information is based on medium-size (20 oz/567 g) drinks.

EXERCISE

Watch your liquid calories! You'll need to bike at a moderate speed for 1.5 hours to burn the 820 calories in the medium Cool Mocha Julius.

ALSO LOSE

PREMIUM FRUIT SMOOTHIES:
Tropi-Colada
› **490** calories
› **77** g sugar
› **102** g carbohydrates

JULIUS VS. COFFEE:
Cool Cappuccino "Moo Latte"
› **710** calories
› **15** g fat
  (**13** g saturated)
› **104** g sugar

JULIUS JUICE:
Triple Berry Juice
› **500** calories
› **9** g fat
  (**7** g saturated)
› **95** g sugar

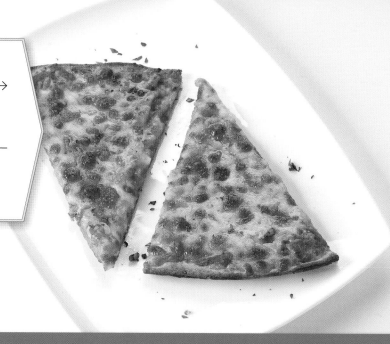

CHOOSE IT

→

QUATTRO CHEESE
(multigrain thin crust, 2 slices)

←

260 CALORIES
9 G FAT (**5** G SATURATED)
300 MG SODIUM

PANAGO

"Panago Pizza's philosophy—"Be bold. Dream fresh."—has brought the restaurant to over 175 locations across Canada, predominantly in B.C. and Alberta. Panago is all about creating fresh, nutritious, chef-inspired food. I have never seen such a wide and delicious-sounding variety of pizza offerings. Healthy options include thin crust with less carbs, low-fat sauces, and healthy proteins. Detailed nutritional information is provided online.

Why choose it? "Four cheeses" sounds like this pizza would be higher in calories and fat, but the thin crust and tomato sauce saves the day here. The nutritional information is based on two slices of medium pizza.

→

ALSO CHOOSE

CHICKEN PIZZA:
Chicken Fajita
› **320** calories
› **10** g fat
  (**6** g saturated)
› **560** g
  carbohydrates

BEEF PIZZA:
Beef Taco
(multigrain
thin crust)
› **320** calories
› **14** g fat
  (**5** g saturated)
› **500** mg sodium

DIPS:
BBQ Sauce
› **35** calories
› **0** g fat
› **290** mg sodium

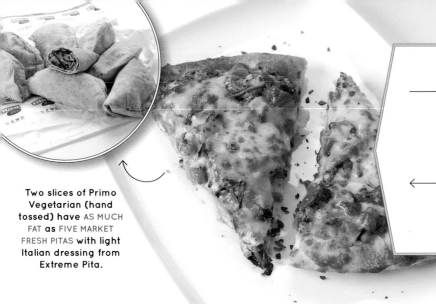

LOSE IT

PRIMO VEGETARIAN
(hand-tossed, 2 slices)

440 CALORIES
18 G FAT (**4** G SATURATED)
480 MG SODIUM

Two slices of Primo Vegetarian (hand tossed) have AS MUCH FAT as FIVE MARKET FRESH PITAS with light Italian dressing from Extreme Pita.

PANAGO

Why lose it? Even though this is vegetarian, the thicker pizza crust and pesto sauce has nearly double the calories and fat of the tomato sauce and thin crust. The nutritional information is based on two slices of medium pizza.

ALSO LOSE

CHICKEN PIZZA:
Chicken Club
› **520** calories
› **24** g fat
  (**6** g saturated)
› **680** mg sodium

BEEF PIZZA:
Steak Mushroom Melt
› **580** calories
› **30** g fat
  (**9** g saturated)
› **920** mg sodium

DIPS:
Chipotle Cilantro
› **140** calories
› **15** g fat
  (**0** g saturated)
› **135** mg sodium

NUTRITION

The crust of a pizza, not just the toppings, can make a difference in calories when you're consuming more than one slice. The Primo Vegetarian has a thin-crust option with 180 calories, a hand-tossed option with 220 calories, a multigrain option with 210 calories and a multigrain thin-crust option with 170 calories. Your best choice would be to select the multigrain thin crust with no extra cheese!

CHOOSE IT

→

FARMER'S OMELETTE

←

1,460 CALORIES
81 G FAT (**29** G SATURATED)
11 G SUGAR
3,320 MG SODIUM

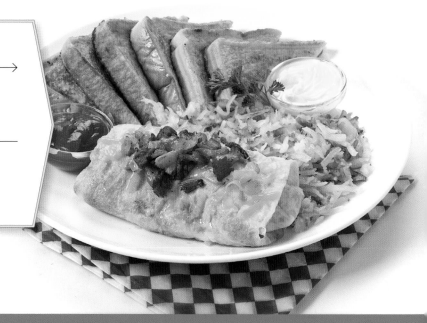

PERKINS RESTAURANT & BAKER

Originally known as Perkins Pancake House, Perkins has been serving diner-style classics since 1958. Today, with 440 full-service family restaurants in the U.S. and Canada, Perkins has a menu that includes over 90 breakfast, lunch, dinner, snack and dessert items. The baked goods are baked on the premises, and the omelettes, buttermilk pancakes, salads and melt sandwiches are all popular with customers. Perkins's website has an excellent nutritional analysis section, which includes everything that comes on the plate, not just the main component of the dish.

Why choose it? This meal, with three eggs, bacon, sausage, sautéed onions, green peppers, cheddar cheese, whipped butter, bread and hash browns is almost a full day's worth of calories, more than a day's worth of fat and almost two days' worth of sodium. But it's the lesser of two evils when compared with Granny's Country Omelette. Make it a birthday breakfast, once a year!

→

ALSO CHOOSE

SANDWICHES & WRAPS:
French Dip Sandwich
(including jus)
› **930** calories
› **51** g fat
   (**13** g saturated)
› **2,580** mg sodium

SALAD:
BLT Chicken Breast Salad
(including ranch dressing)
› **790** calories
› **45** g fat
   (**15** g saturated)
› **1,840** mg sodium

CHILDREN'S MEAL:
Grilled Cheese
(not including fruit cup or butter)
› **370** calories
› **19** g fat
   (**10** g saturated)
› **6** g sugar
› **940** mg sodium

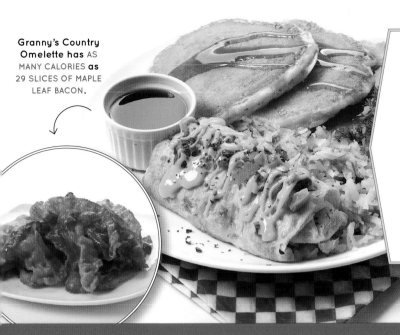

Granny's Country Omelette has AS MANY CALORIES as 29 SLICES OF MAPLE LEAF BACON.

LOSE IT

GRANNY'S COUNTRY OMELETTE

2,060 CALORIES
81 G FAT (**23** G SATURATED)
6,050 MG SODIUM
53 G SUGAR

ERKINS RESTAURANT & BAKERY

Why lose it? Analyzing Perkins's menu items is no easy task, as so many sides are included with the main meal. Just reading the description for this meal (three eggs, ham, onions, cheese, cheese sauce, hash browns, pancakes, syrup, butter) will make you feel you've put on weight! The whole thing adds up to over one day's calorie and fat intake and four days' sodium.

NUTRITION

Eggs are a good source of protein, iron and vitamin A, but they do contain saturated fat and cholesterol in the yolk. Eggs have about 75 calories, 5 g of fat and 250 mg cholesterol. You should be consuming about 320 mg of cholesterol a day, which explains the controversy about excess egg consumption. Egg whites are cholesterol free, and one egg white has only 15 calories, with no fat or cholesterol. Substitute two egg whites for each whole egg in a recipe, or use an egg substitute, which has 80 percent less fat and cholesterol than a regular egg. If you enjoy having more than one egg per day, this is a healthier choice.

ALSO LOSE

SANDWICHES & WRAPS:
The Buffalo Wrap
(including blue cheese dressing)
› **1,460** calories
› **98** g fat
  (**25** g saturated)
› **5,270** mg sodium

SALAD:
Honey Mustard Chicken Crunch Salad
› **1,220** calories
› **83** g fat
  (**21** g saturated)
› **2,510** mg sodium

CHILDREN'S MEAL:
Dollar Pancakes
(including syrup, butter)
› **830** calories
› **26** g fat
  (**8** g saturated)
› **87** g sugar
› **1,310** mg sodium

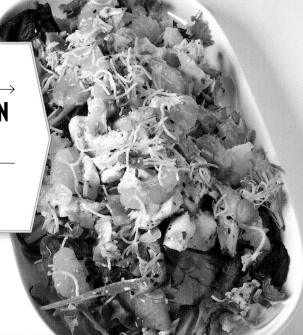

CHOOSE IT

→

CHINESE CHICKEN SALAD

←

660 CALORIES
25 G FAT (**5** G SATURATED)
760 MG SODIUM

PICKLE BARREL

Pickle Barrel is a Canadian establishment that opened its doors in 1971 with an 85-seat diner-style restaurant and has expanded to 12 locations. The restaurants all still adhere to the mission of offering great product and excellent service at superb value. I have been a nutritional consultant with PB for over six years and have created feature menus that are nutritionally balanced. The nutritionals are on the website, along with a gluten-free menu and a healthy menu for children.

Why choose it? Simple unadulterated chicken breast and a plum dressing give you a better nutritional lunch with close to half the calories and sodium and close to a third of the fat as Freddy's Tuna Salad. You even get rice noodles and crisp wontons.

→

ALSO CHOOSE

SANDWICH VS. TACOS:
Jumbo Clubhouse Sandwich
› **530** calories
› **15** g fat
  (**5** g saturated)
› **1,460** mg sodium

APPETIZER:
Mozzarella Sticks
› **490** calories
› **27** g fat
  (**16** g saturated)
› **3,510** mg sodium

PASTA:
Spaghetti & Giant Meatball Pasta
› **810** calories
› **31** g fat
  (**9** g saturated)
› **1,020** mg sodium

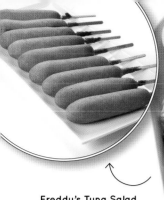

Freddy's Tuna Salad
is EQUIVALENT IN FAT
to NINE Pogo
CORN DOGS.

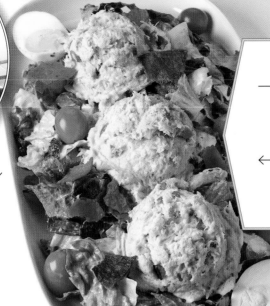

PICKLE BARREL

Why lose it? Tuna salad is often billed as healthy, but when the canned tuna is packed in oil and then mixed with high-fat mayonnaise, it's not a wise choice for the calorie conscious. Add deep-fried tortilla crisps, an egg and an oil-based honey mustard dressing, and you're looking at three-quarters of a day's worth of calories and over a day's worth of fat and sodium.

ALSO LOSE

SANDWICH VS. TACOS:
Fish Tacos
› **1,130** calories
› **72** g fat
   (**19** g saturated)
› **1,340** mg sodium

APPETIZER:
Sweet Potato Fries
› **870** calories
› **61** g fat
   (**6** g saturated)
› **1,950** mg sodium

PASTA:
Chicken Pesto Fettuccine
› **1,220** calories
› **75** g fat
   (**41** g saturated)
› **1,190** mg sodium

HEALTH WARNING

Tuna is a nutritious fish, but when its canned in oil the calories and fat are much higher. Select tuna packed in water. Four oz (113 g) of tuna packed in oil contains 140 calories and 6 g of fat. Four oz of tuna packed in water has only 90 calories and 0.5 g fat. Once you add mayonnaise to a tuna salad, you can see why a tuna sandwich takes you into dangerous nutrient territory!

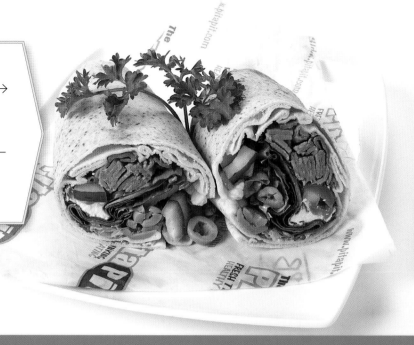

CHOOSE IT

ROAST BEEF PITA
(9 inch/23 cm)

428 CALORIES
11 G FAT
2,417 MG SODIUM

PITA PIT

The Pita Pit says no to high-fat, high-carb, high-sodium junk food and yes to good food served fresh and fast. Opened in 1995 in Kingston, the owners wanted a healthier alternative to the traditional sandwich market. Within two years, the restaurant had expanded across Canada and into the U.S. with over 220 locations. These Lebanese-style pita sandwiches are packed with fresh vegetables, grilled meats and zesty sauces. There is detailed nutrient analysis on the website; the calories and fat are quite low.

Why choose it? Roast beef is a great lean protein for a pita. This option (on a whole-wheat pita, with green olives, lettuce, onions, pineapple and feta) has almost 300 fewer calories and 25 g less fat than the fatty barbecue ribs pita.

ALSO CHOOSE

PITA:
Ham Whole Wheat Pita
(large, 9 inch/23 cm, including green olives, pineapple, baba ghanouj)
› **422** calories
› **11** g fat
› **1,980** mg sodium

SALAD:
Caesar
(large, 164 g)
› **160** calories
› **9** g fat
› **580** mg sodium

BREAKFAST PITA:
Ham 'n' Eggs
(131 g)
› **230** calories
› **8** g fat
› **1,010** mg sodium

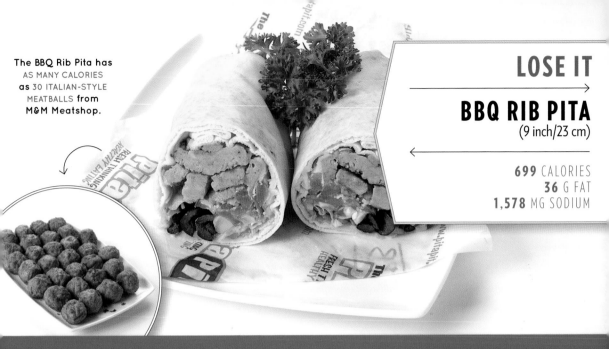

The BBQ Rib Pita has AS MANY CALORIES as 30 ITALIAN-STYLE MEATBALLS from M&M Meatshop.

BBQ RIB PITA
(9 inch/23 cm)

699 CALORIES
36 G FAT
1,578 MG SODIUM

PITA PIT

Why lose it? Pita Pit can be a very healthy "pit stop" if you select wisely. But this barbecue ribs white pita (with olives and cheddar) is not a good choice. This pita accounts for almost half your daily calorie and fat intake and a day's worth of sodium.

ALSO LOSE

PITA:
Gyro White Pita
(large, 9 inches/ 23 cm, including mushrooms, olives, secret sauce)
› **672** calories
› **42** g fat
› **1,418** mg sodium

SALAD:
Garden Salad
(large, 378 g)
› **310** calories
› **23** g fat
› **500** mg sodium

BREAKFAST PITA:
Meat the Day
(139 g)
› **440** calories
› **30** g fat
› **1,020** mg sodium

HEALTH WARNING

Ribs are the fattiest cut of pork. One serving in a restaurant is usually a 1 lb (500 g) rack, which has 1,440 calories, 86 g of fat and 32 g of saturated fat. This adds up to an entire day's worth of calories and more than a day's worth of fat and saturated fat. Compare this to an 8 oz (226 g) pork rib chop, which has only 490 calories, 20 g fat and 8 g of saturated fat. An 8 oz (226 g) serving of pork tenderloin has only 360 calories, 10 g of fat and 2 g of saturated fat.

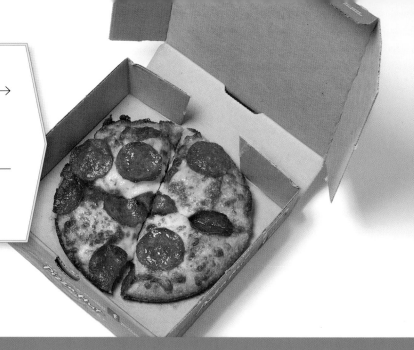

CHOOSE IT

→

PEPPERONI
(personal size, 6 inches/15 cm, multigrain crust)

←

510 CALORIES
17 G FAT (**7** G SATURATED)
790 MG SODIUM

PIZZA HUT

The Pizza Hut legacy began in 1958. Today, there are over 10,000 Pizza Hut locations worldwide, and the company is a subsidiary of Yum Brands, one of the largest restaurant chains in the world. There is a variety of specialty pizzas and crusts, including hand-tossed, thick, stuffed and thin crust. The Eating Well menu offers four multigrain pizzas and two whole-grain pastas. The website has a detailed nutritional section, but you have to remember the name and size of your pizza—there are over 200 pizza options!

Why choose it? You're getting protein in the form of pepperoni, and with the multigrain crust you're getting half the fat and 230 fewer calories than with the personal-size Meat Lover's Pizza.

→

ALSO CHOOSE

PIZZAS:
Cheese Lover's
(12 inches/30 cm, thin crispy crust, 1 slice)
› **240** calories
› **10** g fat
   (**4** g saturated)
› **470** mg sodium

PASTA:
Spaghetti Bolognese
(including meat sauce and cheese)
› **770** calories
› **24** g fat
   (**4** g saturated)
› **1,290** mg sodium

SALAD:
Warm Spinach Salad
› **410** calories
› **29** g fat
   (**5** g saturated)
› **1,080** mg sodium

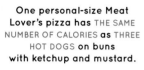

One personal-size Meat Lover's pizza has THE SAME NUMBER OF CALORIES as THREE HOT DOGS on buns with ketchup and mustard.

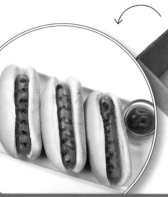

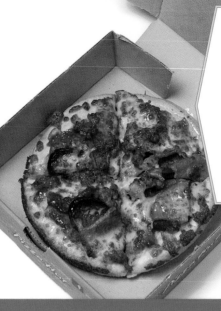

PIZZA HUT

Why lose it? Even a personal pizza can be dangerous when it has "Meat Lovers" in the name. With six different fatty and high-sodium meats, you're getting half of your daily calories, half a day's fat and three-quarters of your daily recommended sodium in this small pizza.

ALSO LOSE

PIZZAS:
Cheese Lover's
(12 inches/30 cm, stuffed crust, 1 slice)
› **420** calories
› **17** g fat
  (**8** g saturated)
› **580** mg sodium

PASTA:
Chicken Pomodoro
(including cream sauce)
› **1,200** calories
› **69** g fat
  (**7** g saturated)
› **2,940** mg sodium

SALAD:
Greek Salad
› **616** calories
› **52** g fat
  (**10** g saturated)
› **1,472** mg sodium

HEALTH WARNING

Stuffed pizza crusts are getting more and more common these days. But the crust can make a huge difference. For example, one slice of a large (14 inch) Pizza Hut Meat Lover's Pizza with stuffed crust has 480 calories, 22 g of fat and 760 mg sodium. Without the stuffed crust, there are only 310 calories, 15 g of fat and 390 mg of sodium.

CHOOSE IT

→

SAUSAGE SANDWICH

←

580 CALORIES
22 G FAT (**5** G SATURATED)
2,350 MG SODIUM

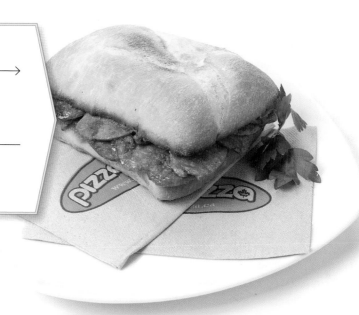

PIZZA PIZZA

Pizza Pizza is a Canadian franchise, which first opened its doors in 1967 in Toronto. There are now over 600 locations, mostly in Ontario and Quebec. In Ontario alone, Pizza Pizza receives over 29 million orders annually! The website includes very detailed nutritionals, an ingredient list and an allergen list. Pizza Pizza's healthy choices include whole wheat multigrain dough, vegan dough and gluten-free toppings and dough; none of the products contain MSG, and trans-fats were removed from the menu in 2004.

Why choose it? The ciabatta bun has almost 300 fewer calories and half the fat of the panzerotti dough. Although sausage is fatty, the total sandwich still has fewer calories and less than half the fat of the Cheese and Pepperoni Panzerotti.

→

ALSO CHOOSE

MEAT PIZZA:
New York Pepperoni
(2 medium slices)
› **420** calories
› **16** g fat
  (**6** g saturated)
› **1,040** mg sodium

PASTA:
Penne Bolognese
› **440** calories
› **9** g fat
  (**2** g saturated)
› **770** mg sodium

WINGS:
Classic Wings
(approximately 6 wings, including chipotle sauce)
› **415** calories
› **26** g fat
  (**7** g saturated)
› **1,485** mg sodium

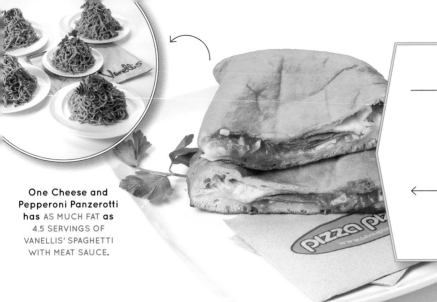

One Cheese and Pepperoni Panzerotti has AS MUCH FAT as 4.5 SERVINGS OF VANELLIS' SPAGHETTI WITH MEAT SAUCE.

LOSE IT

CHEESE & PEPPERONI PANZEROTTI

850 CALORIES
46 G FAT (**20** G SATURATED)
1,890 MG SODIUM

PIZZA PIZZA

Why lose it? A panzerotti is just another name for a closed, filled, often deep-fried pizza. This one has loads of hidden cheese and pepperoni. You're getting about half your daily calories, three-quarters of your daily fat and over a day's worth of sodium.

ALSO LOSE

MEAT PIZZA:
Meat Supreme
(2 medium slices)
› **540** calories
› **24** g fat
  (**9** g saturated)
› **1,620** mg sodium

PASTA:
Cheese Tortolloni Alfredo
› **710** calories
› **41** g fat
  (**24** g saturated)
› **2,040** mg sodium

WINGS:
Crispy Breaded Wings
(approximately 6 wings, including BBQ sauce)
› **800** calories
› **50** g fat
  (**12** g saturated)
› **2,240** mg sodium

WEIGHT LOSS

If you choose the Italian Sausage Sandwich and lose the Cheese and Pepperoni Panzerotti twice a week for one year, you will save yourself 540 calories each week, which works out to a weight loss of 8 lb (4 kg), without having to change anything else in your diet or lifestyle.

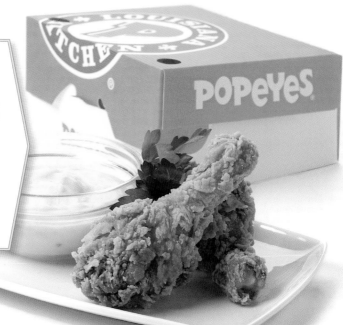

ORIGINAL CHICKEN COMBO (LEGS)
(including mashed potatoes)

430 CALORIES
22 G FAT (**10** G SATURATED)
1,510 MG SODIUM

POPEYES LOUISIANA KITCHEN

"Popeyes" is named after the detective Popeye Doyle, from the movie *The French Connection*, not Popeye the Sailor Man! The cuisine is inspired by Louisiana's Cajun and Creole heritage. Popeyes opened its first franchise restaurant in Baton Rouge in 1972 and has since merged with Church's Chicken. Popeyes went global in 1984, with its first international franchise opening in Toronto. Today, there are locations in 21 countries. The website's nutritional analysis is easy to read.

Why choose it? The two breaded chicken legs have slightly less meat than thighs, and therefore they also have fewer calories and less fat. Choosing mashed potatoes instead of fries saves you 150 calories and 10 g of fat.

ALSO CHOOSE

BIG EASYS:
Naked BBQ Chicken Po-Boy Sandwich
> **340** calories
> **7** g fat
  (**1** g saturated)
> **1,030** mg sodium

SIDES 1:
Cajun Rice
(large, 369 g, including salt dressing, meat sauce)
> **510** calories
> **15** g fat
  (**6** g saturated)
> **1,590** mg sodium

SIDES 2:
Macaroni & Cheese
(large, 469 g)
> **600** calories
> **21** g fat
  (**11** g saturated)
> **1,470** mg sodium

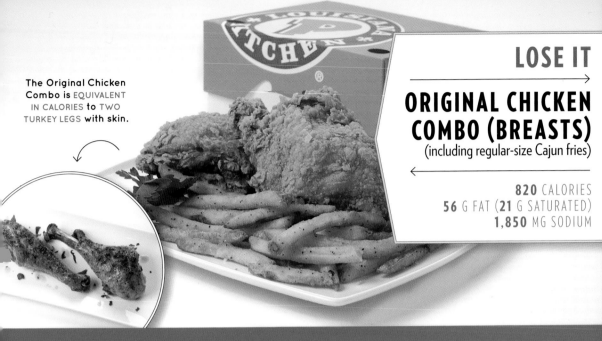

The Original Chicken Combo is EQUIVALENT IN CALORIES to TWO TURKEY LEGS with skin.

LOSE IT →

ORIGINAL CHICKEN COMBO (BREASTS)
(including regular-size Cajun fries)

820 CALORIES
56 G FAT (**21** G SATURATED)
1,850 MG SODIUM

POPEYES LOUISIANA KITCHEN

Why lose it? Nothing but breaded and deep-fried chicken here (two thighs), and with the side order of regular-size Cajun fries you've got over half a day's worth of calories and a day's worth of fat and sodium.

ALSO LOSE

BIG EASYS:

Shrimp Po-Boy Sandwich
› **690** calories
› **42** g fat
  (**13** g saturated)
› **2,156** mg sodium

SIDES 1:

Red Beans & Rice
(large, 438 g)
› **690** calories
› **42** g fat
  (**12** g saturated)
› **1,740** mg sodium

SIDES 2:

Onion Rings
(large, 18 pieces)
› **830** calories
› **56** g fat
  (**25** g saturated)
› **1,370** mg sodium

HEALTH WARNING

Popeyes website shows you the difference in nutrients between eating the skin and crust of the chicken versus removing it. My opinion is that if you're already going into a deep-fried chicken restaurant, you're probably not interesting in removing the "good" stuff. For example, the breaded and fried chicken thigh has 280 calories, 20 g of fat and 710 mg of sodium. When you remove the breaded skin you only have 80 calories, 2 g of fat and 230 mg of sodium. Use some will power, and you'll save yourself a ton of calories, fat and sodium!

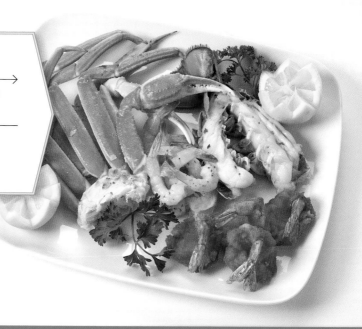

RED LOBSTER

Red Lobster is a seafood chain that opened in the U.S. in 1968; today there are 690 locations in the U.S., several in Canada and one in the United Arab Emirates. With fish and seafood an integral part of a healthy diet, Red Lobster resonates with customers today. Fresh fish is served daily. The chain is known for it Signature Combinations as well as their Cheddar Bay Biscuits. There is a "Light House" menu with items fewer than 500 calories. Nutritional information is available online, but remember to add the sides and sauces.

Why choose it? Ultimate Feast may sound indulgent, but the steamed seafood (lobster tail, snow crab legs, garlic shrimp) with some breaded and fried shrimp, is a better overall choice than the Admiral's Feast. It's half the calories and more than half the fat, but the sodium is still too high.

→

ALSO CHOOSE

STEAK ENTRÉE:
NY Strip & Rock Lobster Tail
(14 oz/397 g, including mashed potatoes)
› **590** calories
› **29** g fat
  (**12** g saturated)
› **1,700** mg sodium

SEASIDE STARTERS:
Fire-Grilled Shrimp Bruschetta
› **650** calories
› **26** g fat
  (**4** g saturated)
› **2,380** mg sodium

CLAM CHOWDER:
Manhattan Clam Chowder
(1 bowl)
› **160** calories
› **2** g fat
  (**1** g saturated)
› **1,425** mg sodium

↓

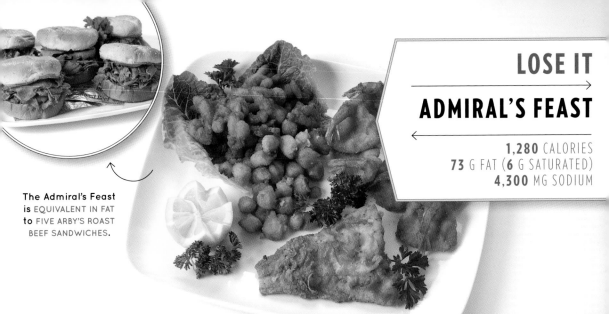

LOSE IT

ADMIRAL'S FEAST

1,280 CALORIES
73 G FAT (**6** G SATURATED)
4,300 MG SODIUM

The Admiral's Feast is EQUIVALENT IN FAT to FIVE ARBY'S ROAST BEEF SANDWICHES.

RED LOBSTER

Why lose it? No admiral would be fit for service after eating this plate of oily deep-fried fish! "Lightly breaded" doesn't begin to describe this meal (shrimp, bay scallops, clam strips and fried haddock), which has three-quarters of a day's worth of calories, over a day's worth of fat and almost three days' worth of sodium.

HEALTH WARNING

Much of today's fish is either endangered or contains mercury and other toxins that are dangerous to our health. There are a couple of great websites, Seafoodwatch.org and Oceanwise.ca, that list sustainable seafood choices, and provide advice on which seafood to avoid, which species are overfished or fished in ways that hurt the environment and which have high levels of contaminants. The Super Green List recommends fish that is good for human health and whose fishing practices do not harm the ocean.

ALSO LOSE

STEAK ENTRÉE:
Steak, Lobster & Shrimp Oscar
(14 oz/397 g, including asparagus, sauce, potatoes)
› **1,120** calories
› **72** g fat
   (**33** g saturated)
› **2,670** mg sodium

SEASIDE STARTERS:
Shrimp Nachos
› **1090** calories
› **64** g fat
   (**19** g saturated)
› **1,680** mg sodium

CLAM CHOWDER:
New England Clam Chowder
(1 bowl)
› **480** calories
› **34** g fat
   (**20** g saturated)
› **1,390** mg sodium

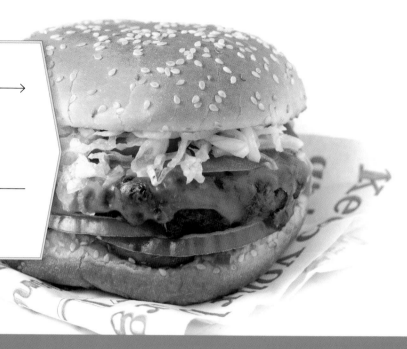

→

CHOOSE IT

RED ROBIN GOURMET CHEESEBURGER

790 CALORIES
45 G FAT (**18** G SATURATED)
1,530 MG SODIUM

RED ROBIN

Red Robin Gourmet Burgers has been a burger expert since it first opened its doors in Seattle in 1969. It now has over 450 restaurants across the U.S. and Canada. It serves innovative, gourmet beef burgers, turkey burgers, vegan burgers and chicken sandwiches, as well as salads, entrées, chilies, chowders, steak fries and bottomless beverages. Red Robin believes in quality and "honest to goodness" ingredients, meaning that the fries are cooked in zero trans-fat oil and the ingredients are fresh. The restaurant website includes easy-to-read nutritionals.

Why choose it? This gourmet burger has almost 300 fewer calories and almost 30 grams of fat less than the Royal Burger. The only difference is the lack of egg and bacon. You even get to enjoy cheddar cheese and creamy mayo.

ALSO CHOOSE

CHICKEN BURGERS:
Mediterranean Chicken Burger
› **550** calories
› **19** g fat
  (**7** g saturated)
› **1,760** mg sodium

WRAPS AND SANDWICHES:
Mediterranean Wrap
› **640** calories
› **26** g fat
  (**9** g saturated)
› **2,010** mg sodium

CHILDREN'S MENU:
Cheesy Mac 'n' Cheese
(including baby carrots, ranch dressing)
› **370** calories
› **22** g fat
  (**8** g saturated)
› **1,310** mg sodium

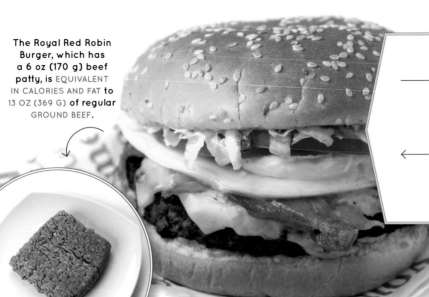

The Royal Red Robin Burger, which has a 6 oz (170 g) beef patty, is EQUIVALENT IN CALORIES AND FAT to 13 OZ (369 G) of regular GROUND BEEF.

LOSE IT →

ROYAL RED ROBIN BURGER

1,050 CALORIES
72 G FAT (**24** G SATURATED)
1,910 MG SODIUM

RED ROBIN

Why lose it? You get a quadruple whammy of calories, fat, saturated fat and sodium in this not-so-"Royal" burger! There is three-quarters of a day's worth of calories and more than a day's worth of fat and sodium in the fried egg, bacon, processed cheese and mayo—a coronary time-bomb!

ALSO LOSE

CHICKEN BURGERS:
Whiskey River BBQ Chicken Burger
› **840** calories
› **51** g fat
   (**13** g saturated)
› **1,480** mg sodium

WRAPS AND SANDWICHES:
Whiskey River BBQ Chicken Wrap
› **900** calories
› **44** g fat
   (**17** g saturated)
› **2,180** mg sodium

CHILDREN'S MENU:
Carnival Corn Dog
(including salad, ranch dressing)
› **700** calories
› **55** g fat
   (**12** g saturated)
› **1,170** mg sodium

TRIVIA

Red Robin was originally named Sam's Tavern, after its original owner. Sam sang in a barbershop quartet and could frequently be heard singing a song called "When the Red, Red Robin (Comes Bob, Bob, Bobbin' Along)." He liked the song so much that he eventually changed the name of the restaurant to Sam's Red Robin; now it's known simply as Red Robin.

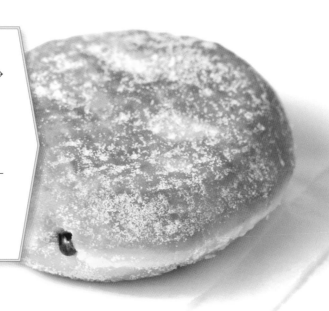

STRAWBERRY WHITE YEAST DONUT

250 CALORIES
9 G FAT (**4** G SATURATED)
11 G SUGAR
38 G CARBOHYDRATES

ROBIN'S DONUTS

Robin's Donuts opened its doors in 1975 in Thunder Bay, Ontario, has grown to 130 locations across Canada and is one of the top-grossing donut chains in western Canada. It is typically open 24 hours a day/seven days a week. Aside from donuts, it offers hot and cold beverages, including fair trade coffee, handmade baked goods, breakfast items, soups and sandwiches. Nutritional facts are clearly listed online.

Why choose it? When a donut has half the calories, fat and carbs and one-quarter of the sugar of the healthy-sounding Carrot Muffin, you can occasionally allow yourself to indulge.

ALSO CHOOSE

DONUT VS. MUFFIN:
Sour Cream Glazed Donut
› **300** calories
› **8** g fat
  (**4** g saturated)
› **54** g carbohydrates
› **33** g sugar

SANDWICH:
Classic Club
› **340** calories
› **9** g fat
  (**2** g saturated)
› **1,240** mg sodium

BREAKFAST SANDWICH:
Bacon, Egg & Cheese Brekwich
› **410** calories
› **24** g fat
  (**10** g saturated)
› **1,140** mg sodium

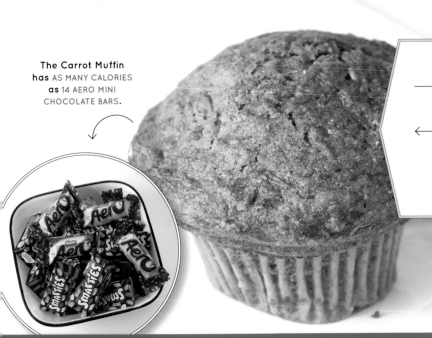

The Carrot Muffin **has** AS MANY CALORIES **as** 14 AERO MINI CHOCOLATE BARS.

LOSE IT →

CARROT MUFFIN

560 CALORIES
23 G FAT (**2** G SATURATED)
83 G CARBOHYDRATES
48 G SUGAR

ROBIN'S DONUTS

Why lose it? We'd like to think that a vegetable-based muffin is good for us. But this one muffin (filled with oil or shortening and excess sugar) has one-third of your daily calories, almost half a day's worth of fat and a day's worth of sugar, approximately 12 tsp (60 mL)!

ALSO LOSE

DONUT VS. MUFFIN:
Chocolate Chip Muffin
› **510** calories
› **24** g fat
   (**4** g saturated)
› **69** g carbohydrates
› **35** g sugar

SANDWICH:
Chunky Chicken Salad Sandwich
› **500** calories
› **27** g fat
   (**2** g saturated)
› **860** mg sodium

BREAKFAST SANDWICH:
Sausage, Egg & Cheese Brekwich
› **510** calories
› **32** g fat
   (**13** g saturated)
› **1,390** mg sodium

HOME COOKING

Fruit- or vegetable-stuffed muffins sound so healthy, but muffins are basically just small cakes with excess oil and sugar. And lest you think low-fat muffins are much better, they often have more sugar to compensate for the lack of oil. If you bake your own muffins at home, try reducing the sugar in the recipe by 25 percent (or use Splenda) and the oil by as much as 50 percent, replacing it with light sour cream, yogurt or pureed banana. You'll be surprised by how little these healthy switches affect the flavour.

CHOOSE IT

→

MOCCACHINO
(medium, 16 oz/454 g, skim milk,
not including whipped cream)

←

300 CALORIES
5 G FAT (**4** G SATURATED)
42 G SUGAR

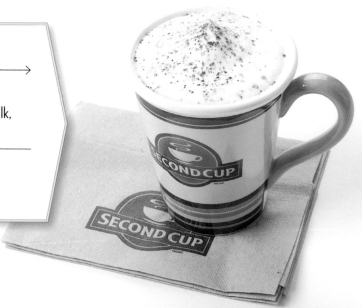

SECOND CUP

Established in 1975, Second Cup is the largest Canadian specialty coffee franchise and retailer, with 360 cafés across Canada and 50 international cafés. Most of the coffee beans used are exclusive to Second Cup and come from some of the world's best coffee estates The company website has an excellent nutrition section, but remember to check the boxes for size, milk type and whipped cream. The nutritional information given here is for medium (16 oz/454 g) drinks.

Why choose it? With 120 fewer calories than the White Mocha and 19 g less fat, the Moccachino, with some chocolate, is a delicious and more acceptable way to drink your calories. Semi-sweet chocolate has fewer calories and less fat per ounce.

ALSO CHOOSE

→

SPECIALTIES:	TEA LATTE:	LEMONADE:
Matcha Green Chiller	**London Fog**	**Sparkling Green Tea Lemonade**
(two percent milk)	(skim milk)	› **100** calories
› **190** calories	› **290** calories	› **0.1** g fat
› **3** g fat	› **8** g fat	› **25** g carbohydrates
(**2** g saturated)	(**5** g saturated)	› **24** g sugar
› **33** g carbohydrates	› **40** g carbohydrates	
› **33** g sugar	› **20** g sugar	

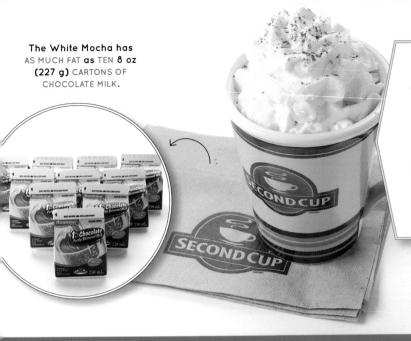

The White Mocha has AS MUCH FAT as TEN **8 oz (227 g)** CARTONS OF CHOCOLATE MILK.

WHITE MOCHA
(medium, 16 oz/454 g, two percent milk, including whipped cream)

460 CALORIES
24 G FAT (**17** G SATURATED)
43 G SUGAR

SECOND CUP

Why lose it? The whipped cream and white chocolate syrup make this more of a dessert than a coffee. With almost one-third of your daily calories and half your daily fat, think of this as a special treat rather than a regular indulgence.

ALSO LOSE

SPECIALTIES:
Classic Hot Chocolate
(skim milk)
› **340** calories
› **6** g fat
  (**5** g saturated)
› **59** g carbohydrates
› **49** g sugar

TEA LATTE:
Chai Latte
(two percent milk)
› **420** calories
› **12** g fat
  (**9** g saturated)
› **64** g carbohydrates
› **44** g sugar

LEMONADE:
Strawberry Lemonade Chiller
› **370** calories
› **0** g fat
› **93** g carbohydrates
› **90** g sugar

NUTRITION

For years, coffee has gotten bad press with respect to health. It's been blamed for everything from causing heart disease and cancer to stunting our growth! But the good news is that drinking coffee in moderation is actually good for us. Recent studies show no correlation between coffee and an increased risk of cancer or heart disease. Coffee has even been shown to help stave off Parkinson's disease, type 2 diabetes and liver cancer, and it's loaded with antioxidants. Just watch out for coffee beverages that contain an excess of higher-fat milk, whipped cream and sugar. Keep it to four cups maximum per day.

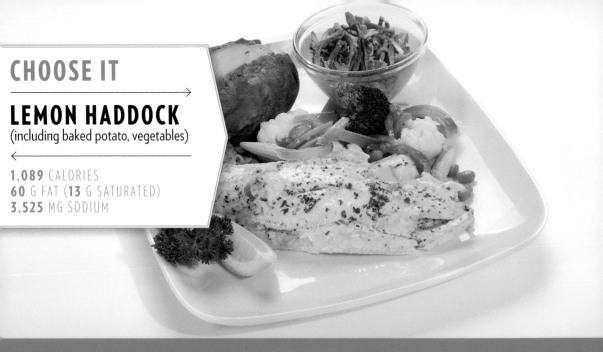

CHOOSE IT →

LEMON HADDOCK
(including baked potato, vegetables)

1,089 CALORIES
60 G FAT (**13** G SATURATED)
3,525 MG SODIUM

SHOELESS JOE'S

Shoeless Joe's opened in Toronto in 1985 and has since expanded across Ontario. The sports-themed restaurant has a casual flair and offers personalized service to its customers. Nutritional information is available online, but careful with the entrées—you might have to add the side-dish nutritionals separately. When it comes to fries, I would recommend substituting the regular french fries with lattice or sweet potato fries. The french fries are over 1,000 calories and have 5,000 mg of sodium!

Why choose it? Pan-seared means lots of oil, but it's better than deep-fried. Still, this dish, with baked potatoes and vegetables, has three-quarters of a day's worth of calories, over a day's worth of fat and two days' worth of sodium.

ALSO CHOOSE

PASTA/GRAINS:
Smoked Mozzarella Ravioli
› **841** calories
› **50** g fat (**22** g saturated)
› **1,521** mg sodium

SANDWICH:
Pulled Pork Sandwich
(including barbecue sauce)
› **513** calories
› **15** g fat (**4** g saturated)
› **912** mg sodium

SALAD:
Mediterranean Salad
(including vegetables, feta, olives, feta dressing)
› **562** calories
› **39** g fat (**12** g saturated)
› **776** mg sodium

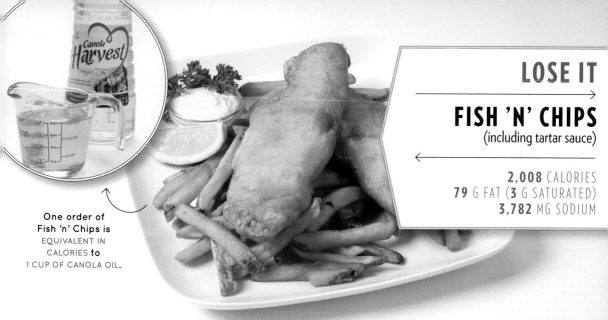

One order of
Fish 'n' Chips is
EQUIVALENT IN
CALORIES to
1 CUP OF CANOLA OIL.

LOSE IT

FISH 'N' CHIPS
(including tartar sauce)

2,008 CALORIES
79 G FAT (**3** G SATURATED)
3,782 MG SODIUM

SHOELESS JOE'S

Why lose it? Fish and chips spells mega calories and fat. Battered and deep-fried fish with tartar sauce and fries is the worst combination possible. Close to one and a half days' worth of calories, three days' worth of fat and almost five days' worth of sodium! Enjoy this dish once a year, if that!

NUTRITION

Excess salt in our diet can increase blood pressure, which can lead to heart disease, stroke and kidney failure. There is also a link between sodium and stomach cancer. Hidden salt is the most dangerous—77 percent of the salt in our diet comes from packed, processed and restaurant foods, 12 percent occurs naturally in foods, 5 percent is added in home cooking and 6 percent is added during our meals—the worst offenders are canned foods, tomato sauces, pickled foods and deli meats.

ALSO LOSE

PASTA/GRAINS:
Chicken Shrimp Quinoa
› **1,685** calories
› **104** g fat
  (**17** g saturated)
› **2,761** mg sodium

SANDWICH:
Chicken Fajita Wrap
(including rice)
› **1,014** calories
› **47** g fat
  (**17** g saturated)
› **1,760** mg sodium

SALAD:
Chipotle Southwest Chicken Salad
(including dressing)
› **1,036** calories
› **74** g fat
  (**9** g saturated)
› **1,920** mg sodium

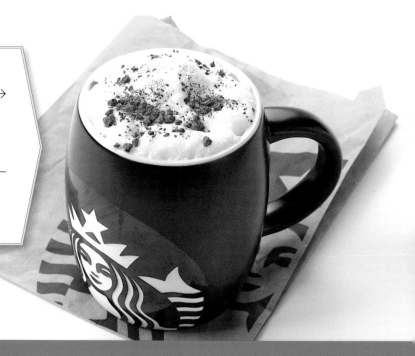

CHOOSE IT

HOT CHOCOLATE
(two percent milk, not including whipped cream)

290 CALORIES
9 G FAT (**5** G SATURATED)
41 G SUGAR

PART 1 STARBUCKS

Starbucks opened its doors as a coffee bean store in 1971 in Seattle's historical Pike Place Market. Howard Schultz became CEO of Starbucks in 1982 and a year later went to Italy, where he was inspired by Italian coffee bars. He came back with the idea of selling coffee and espresso drinks at Starbucks, not just beans. Today there are more than 17,000 Starbucks locations in over 50 countries. The first Starbucks in Canada opened its doors in 1987 in Vancouver. Starbucks sells Americanos, lattes, mochas,

continued on page 134

Why choose it? Losing the whipped cream saves you 80 calories and 7 g of fat, for a better-for-you hot chocolate. If you opt for one percent milk, you can reduce the calories to 240 and the fat to only 2.5 g of fat. Nutritional information for beverages is based on a grande-size drink (16 oz/454 g).

ALSO CHOOSE

ESPRESSO:
Caramel Macchiato
(two percent milk)
› **240** calories
› **7** g fat
  (**3** g saturated)
› **150** mg sodium
› **34** g carbohydrates
› **32** g sugar

FRAPPUCCINO:
Vanilla Bean Crème Frappucino
(non-fat milk)
› **240** calories
› **0.1** g fat
  (**0.1** g saturated)
› **56** g carbohydrates
› **55** g sugar

MUFFINS:
Blueberry Struesel Muffin
› **360** calories
› **11** g fat
  (**6** g saturated)
› **59** g carbohydrates
› **33** g sugar

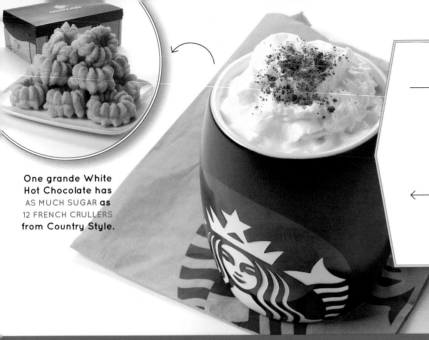

One grande White Hot Chocolate has AS MUCH SUGAR as 12 FRENCH CRULLERS from Country Style.

LOSE IT

WHITE HOT CHOCOLATE
(two percent milk, including whipped cream)

490 CALORIES
19 G FAT (**12** G SATURATED)
62 G SUGAR

STARBUCKS PART 1

Why lose it? The white chocolate is higher in calories, fat and sugar than dark chocolate. With whipped cream you've got almost one-third your daily calories and one and a half days' worth of sugar. Nutritional information for beverages is based on a grande-size drink (16 oz/454 g).

WEIGHT LOSS

If you enjoy the White Hot Chocolate beverage at least three times per week instead of the Hot Chocolate without whipped cream, you'll be looking at a weight gain of 9 lb (4 kg) by the end of the year! Not worth it!

ALSO LOSE

ESPRESSO:
Salted Caramel Mocha
(including whipped cream)
› **420** calories
› **16** g fat
  (**9** g saturated)
› **56** g sugar

FRAPPUCCINO:
Strawberries & Cream
(whole milk, including whipped cream)
› **370** calories
› **15** g fat
  (**9** g saturated)
› **39** g sugar

MUFFINS:
Zucchini Walnut Muffin
› **490** calories
› **28** g fat
  (**2** g saturated)
› **52** g carbohydrates
› **28** g sugar

CHOOSE IT

→

BUTTER CROISSANT

←

380 CALORIES
22 G FAT (**13** G SATURATED)
290 MG SODIUM
39 G CARBOHYDRATES
5 G SUGAR

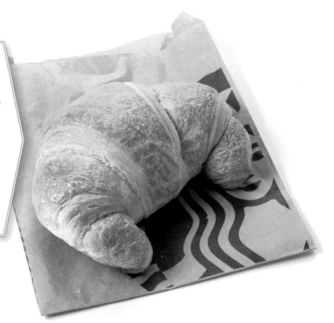

PART 2 STARBUCKS

continued from page 132

cappuccinos, macchiatos, espressos, flavoured iced coffees and its famous Frappuccinos; it also offers fresh food. Starbucks prides itself on being a responsible company. It uses ethical sourcing and responsible growing practices and reduces its environmental foot print through energy and water conservation, recycling and green construction.

Why choose it? Who would believe that a butter croissant is a better selection than a scone? With 170 fewer calories, 7 g less fat and half the carbs, this is definitely a better choice for breakfast on the go. But don't make it a daily habit!

→

ALSO CHOOSE

SNACK PLATE-
BISTRO BOX:
Protein Bistro Box
› **360** calories
› **18** g fat
› **35** g carbohydrates

HOT BREAKFAST:
Ham & Cheddar Artisan Breakfast Sandwich
› **350** calories
› **16** g fat
  (**6** g saturated)
› **790** mg sodium
› **31** g carbohydrates

SNACK:
Chocolate Caramel Pretzel
› **230** calories
› **9** g fat
› **34** g carbohydrates

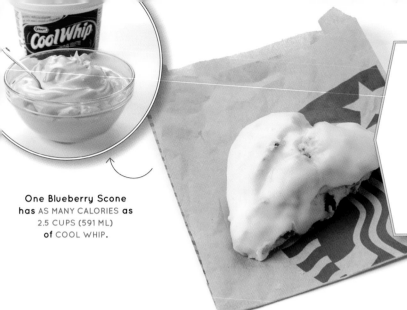

One Blueberry Scone
has AS MANY CALORIES as
2.5 CUPS (591 ML)
of COOL WHIP.

STARBUCKS PART 2

Why lose it? The perennial British baked good looks and tastes quite innocent in terms of calories, fat and sugar. But lo and behold, scones are filled with unhealthy nutrients, including excess sodium.

ALSO LOSE

SNACK PLATE-
BISTRO BOX:
Cheese & Fruit Plate
› **480** calories
› **28** g fat
› **39** g carbohydrates

HOT BREAKFAST:
Sausage & Cheddar Classic Breakfast Sandwich
› **500** calories
› **28** g fat
  (**9** g saturated)
› **920** mg sodium
› **41** g carbohydrates

SNACK:
Chocolate Chip Cookie
› **440** calories
› **21** g fat
› **62** g carbohydrates

TRIVIA

Starbucks is named after the first mate in *Moby-Dick*. The chain has over 11,000 stores in the U.S., over 1,000 in Canada, over 700 in the U.K. and over 150 in Turkey. Overseas stores now account for one-third of the franchise. For a period in the 1990s, Starbucks opened a new store every workday, a pace that continued into the 2000s.

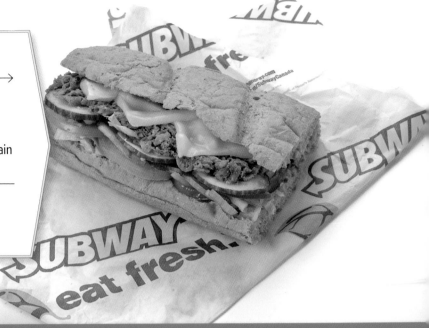

CHOOSE IT →

STEAK AND CHEESE SUB

(6 inches/15 cm, including nine-grain wheat bread, vegetables)

380 CALORIES
9 G FAT (**4** G SATURATED)
1,060 MG SODIUM

SUBWAY

Subway is the world's largest submarine sandwich franchise. It has over 35,000 locations in 98 countries. The first Canadian Subway opened in 1986 in St. John's, Newfoundland. Subway has transformed the fast-food world, offering healthier alternatives to traditionally greasy and fatty fare. The sandwiches are made right in front of customers. A special selection of healthy sandwiches have no more than 7 g of fat, are under 350 calories and are served on a 6 inch (15 cm) nine-grain bread. The website has detailed nutritional information.

Why choose it? I love that steak and cheese is actually better for you than tuna in this case. With close to half the calories and a quarter of the fat, you have a satisfying selection.

ALSO CHOOSE

SANDWICH:
Subway Club
(6 inches/15 cm, including light mayo)
› **415** calories
› **19** g fat
  (**5** g saturated)
› **1,155** mg sodium

BREAKFAST OMELETTE:
Ham & Cheese Omelette Sandwich
› **400** calories
› **14** g fat
  (**5** g saturated)
› **990** mg sodium

MINI SUBS:
Roast Beef Mini Sub
› **190** calories
› **3** g fat
  (**1** g saturated)
› **480** mg sodium

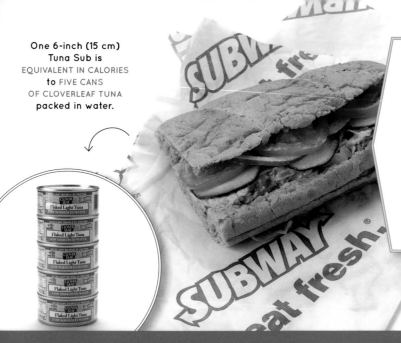

One 6-inch (15 cm) Tuna Sub is EQUIVALENT IN CALORIES to FIVE CANS OF CLOVERLEAF TUNA packed in water.

LOSE IT →

TUNA SUB

(6 inches/15 cm, including nine-grain wheat bread, vegetables, Southwest sauce, light mayo)

620 CALORIES
39 G FAT (**6** G SATURATED)
935 MG SODIUM

SUBWAY

Why lose it? We know tuna as a healthy fish that's lean and filled with Omega-3 fatty acids. But canned tuna is packed in oil and then mixed with high-fat, high-calorie mayonnaise. That's why you're getting three-quarters of your daily recommended calories and fat in one small sandwich, not to mention half your daily sodium.

ALSO LOSE

SANDWICH:
Italian BMT
(6 inches/15 cm, including ranch dressing, house sauce)
› **630** calories
› **39** g fat
   (**10** g saturated)
› **1,610** mg sodium

BREAKFAST OMELETTE:
Sausage & Cheese Omelette Sandwich
› **620** calories
› **37** g fat
   (**14** g saturated)
› **1,290** mg sodium

MINI SUBS:
Tuna Mini Sub
› **270** calories
› **12** g fat
   (**2** g saturated)
› **360** mg sodium

TRIVIA

Jared Fogle, known as the "Subway Guy," became Subway's spokesperson in 2000. He is known for losing 100 lb (45 kg) on what was called the Subway Diet. When the company's sales doubled to $8.2 billion in 2000 and 2001, it was largely attributed to Jared's endorsement. Jared maintained his weight loss for 10 years and retired his old pair of 62-inch (157 cm)-waist pants to a museum. It's reported that he has a net worth of $15 million, thanks to his association with Subway.

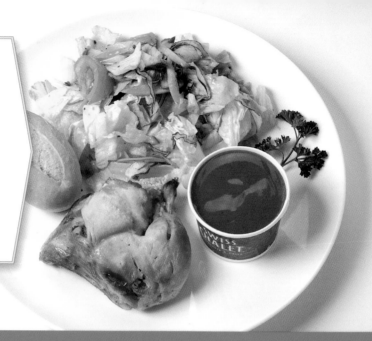

CHOOSE IT

→

QUARTER CHICKEN DINNER

(dark meat without skin, roll, dipping sauce, garden salad, dressing)

←

345 CALORIES
12 G FAT (**3** G SATURATED)
1,365 MG SODIUM

SWISS CHALET

Swiss Chalet is a Canadian family restaurant chain that first opened in Toronto in 1954. Parent company Cara Operations also owns Harvey's, which is why you'll often find the two restaurants sharing one location. Swiss Chalet is all about "real food made fresh by real people." Its specialties are rotisserie chicken based on a Swiss recipe. Nutritional and allergy information is on the website along with a selection of healthy meals featuring the Heart and Stroke Foundation's Health Check seal.

Why choose it? Enjoy the richness of dark meat, but don't eat the skin. Also enjoy the garden salad with its light Italian dressing (instead of a caesar salad) and a roll and dipping sauce, and you've saved yourself over 300 calories, half the fat and one-third of the artery-clogging saturated fat of the Lose It option.

→

ALSO CHOOSE

SANDWICH:
Classic Hot Chicken Sandwich
(white meat, including gravy)
› **520** calories
› **11** g fat
  (**3** g saturated)
› **1,850** mg sodium

SIDES:
Mashed Potatoes
› **150** calories
› **4** g fat
  (**1** g saturated)
› **410** mg sodium

CHILDREN'S MEAL:
Kids Quarter Chicken
(dark meat)
› **240** calories
› **16** g fat
  (**5** g saturated)
› **220** mg sodium

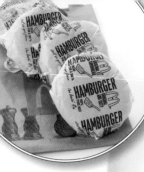

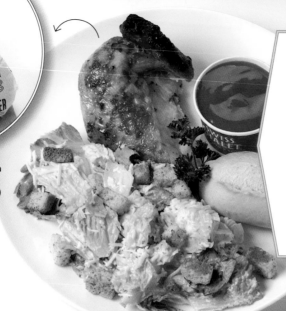

The Quarter Chicken Dinner with white meat (skin included) has the SAME AMOUNT OF FAT as FOUR MCDONALD'S HAMBURGERS.

LOSE IT

QUARTER CHICKEN DINNER
(white meat with skin, roll, dipping sauce, caesar salad, dressing)

655 CALORIES
31 G FAT (**7** G SATURATED)
1,535 MG SODIUM

SWISS CHALET

Why lose it? Even though white chicken meat is generally better for you than dark, the skin adds extra calories and fat. A caesar salad is always more fattening and calorie dense because of the dressing.

ALSO LOSE

SANDWICH:
Rotisserie Chicken Club Wrap
› **710** calories
› **32** g fat
  (**11** g saturated)
› **1,450** mg sodium

SIDES:
Seasoned Rice
› **240** calories
› **3** g fat
  (**0.3** g saturated)
› **830** mg sodium

CHILDREN'S MEAL:
Cheesy Pizza
› **440** calories
› **18** g fat
  (**8** g saturated)
› **840** mg sodium

TRIVIA

To eat the chicken skin or not? That is the question! I would advise not. A 4 oz (113 g) boneless, skinless chicken breast has 118 calories and 1.4 g of fat. Eat the skin and you will consume 188 calories and 11 g of fat. There are 138 calories and 3.2 g of fat in a chicken thigh without skin and 211 calories and 10 g of fat with skin. One chicken wing without skin has 100 calories and 3.2 g of fat, and a wing with skin has 237 calories and 13 g of fat. The skin accounts for over 80 percent of the calories in the chicken.

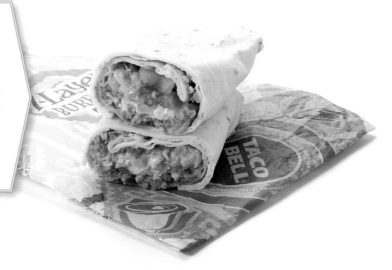

TACO BELL

Taco Bell is an American fast-food chain based in Irvine, California. Serving Mexican food adapted to the American palate, Taco Bell is now in over 26 countries. Founder Glen Bell opened his first restaurant in 1946 in San Bernardino, California. He expanded to selling burgers and eventually tacos, after inventing a new way to fry tacos. The menu offers tacos, burritos, quesadillas and frescoes, considered their healthier choices. Nutritional and allergen information is online.

Why choose it? Go ahead and enjoy some protein-filled steak with loads of vegetables and a low-calorie, low-fat salsa. With half the fat and saturated fat of the Seven-Layer Burrito, this is the better Taco Bell choice.

→

ALSO CHOOSE

TACOS:
Beef Soft Taco Supreme
(including reduced-fat sour cream)
› **210** calories
› **10** g fat
  (**4** g saturated)
› **470** mg sodium

SOFT TACO:
Fresco Chicken Soft Taco
› **170** calories
› **5** g fat
  (**2** g saturated)
› **580** mg sodium

SPECIALTIES:
Mexi Melt
› **280** calories
› **14** g fat
  (**7** g saturated)
› **620** mg sodium

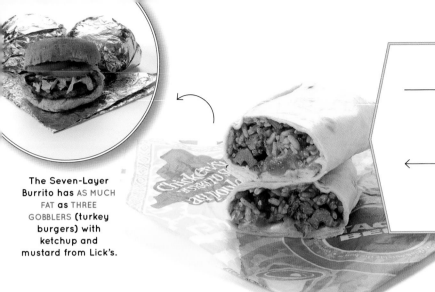

The Seven-Layer Burrito has AS MUCH FAT as THREE GOBBLERS (turkey burgers) with ketchup and mustard from Lick's.

TACO BELL

Why lose it? Anything with seven layers in a Mexican restaurant can't be healthy! Even though this is a vegetarian burrito, the cheddar, jack and mozzarella cheeses, and the rice, beans, sour cream and guacamole all add to the calories, fat and saturated fat.

ALSO LOSE

TACOS:
Cheesy Gordita Crunch
› **500** calories
› **29** g fat
   (**10** g saturated)
› **740** mg sodium

SOFT TACO:
Grilled Steak Soft Taco
› **250** calories
› **14** g fat
   (**4** g saturated)
› **410** mg sodium

SPECIALTIES:
Chicken Quesadilla
› **530** calories
› **28** g fat
   (**12** g saturated)
› **1,170** mg sodium

MENU

Taco Bell's Fresco Menu is excellent if you are watching your calories or fat. The average taco with either beef, chicken or steak is approximately 170 calories, with only 7 g of fat and 400 mg of sodium. Avoid the specialty items such as the Cheesy Gordita Crunch and the Chicken Quesadilla, which has around 500 calories and 25 g of fat, and almost 1,200 mg of sodium!

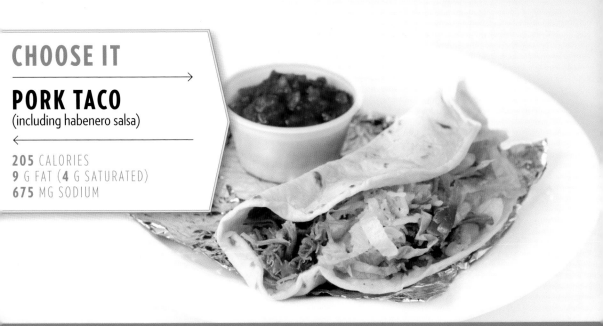

PORK TACO
(including habenero salsa)

205 CALORIES
9 G FAT (**4** G SATURATED)
675 MG SODIUM

TACO DEL MAR

Taco Del Mar is a "fast, fun and delicious alternative to traditional Mexican food." Since opening in Seattle's historical waterfront district in 1992, it is now located in 17 states as well as the provinces of Alberta, British Columbia, Ontario and Saskatchewan. There are over 260 Taco Del Mar locations in all. Its signature meals include fish tacos, quesadillas, enchiladas and Mondo Burritos. The website has clearly laid-out nutritional information, as well as lower-calorie, gluten-free, vegetarian and vegan menus.

Why choose it? The salsa and non-fried pork add up to fewer calories and less fat than the deep-fried Fish Taco with its high-fat sour cream.

ALSO CHOOSE

MONDO BURRITO:
Carne Asada Steak Mondo Burrito
› **820** calories
› **23** g fat
  (**9** g saturated)
› **2,280** mg sodium

SALAD:
Shredded Beef Cabo Salad
(including dressing)
› **420** calories
› **19** g fat
  (**7** g saturated)
› **1,320** mg sodium

CHILDREN'S MEAL:
Kid's Taco Carne Asada Steak
› **190** calories
› **10** g fat
  (**3** g saturated)
› **390** mg sodium

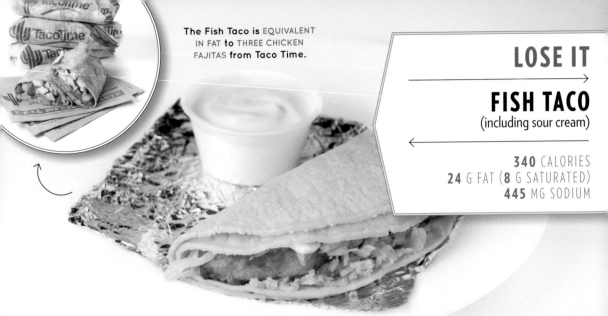

The Fish Taco is EQUIVALENT IN FAT to THREE CHICKEN FAJITAS from Taco Time.

LOSE IT →

FISH TACO
(including sour cream)

340 CALORIES
24 G FAT (**8** G SATURATED)
445 MG SODIUM

TACO DEL MAR

Why lose it? Fish is a lean, heart-healthy protein, but in this taco it's been deep-fried. Add cheese, sour cream and a mayonnaise-based white sauce, and you'll understand where the fat comes from.

ALSO LOSE

MONDO BURRITO:
Fish Mondo Burrito
› **900** calories
› **42** g fat
  (**11** g saturated)
› **2,000** mg sodium

SALAD:
Fish Taco Salad
(including white sauce)
› **840** calories
› **51** g fat
  (**11** g saturated)
› **1,320** mg sodium

CHILDREN'S MEAL:
Kid's Chips & Cheese
› **370** calories
› **21** g fat
  (**8** g saturated)
› **450** mg sodium

NUTRITION

A soft flour tortilla or a small hard taco shell: which is the better choice? A small, 6-inch (15 cm) flour tortilla has 100 calories, 2.5 g of fat and 290 mg of sodium, compared with a hard taco shell, which has 50 calories, 2 g of fat and only 45 mg of sodium. But remember, what goes into the tortilla or taco makes or breaks the meal.

→

CHICKEN FAJITA BURRITO

358 CALORIES
8 G FAT (**4** G SATURATED)
1,090 MG SODIUM
45 G CARBOHYDRATES

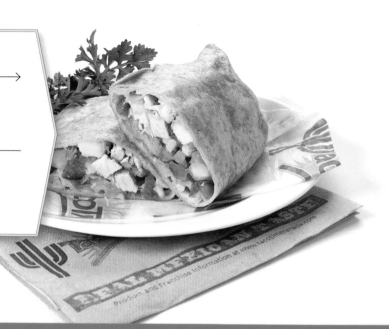

TACO TIME

Taco Time was founded in 1959 in Eugene, Oregon, and launched its first international restaurant in Lethbridge, Alberta. It has since expanded to 300 locations, in Canada, Kuwait and Curacao in the Netherlands Antilles. Canadian outlets are located in British Columbia, Alberta, Saskatchewan, Manitoba and Ontario. The menu includes Mexican favourites such as burritos, tacos, salads, quesadillas, nachos, Mexi-fries, desserts and a kids' menu. The website is quite basic, but it does include good nutritional and allergen information.

Why choose it? This is a healthy choice with the extra veggies, no rice and a low-calorie salsa rather than a mayo-based dressing. You save half the fat and almost 150 calories.

→

ALSO CHOOSE

BURRITO:
Super Beef Burrito
› **451** calories
› **20** g fat
    (**10** g saturated)
› **915** mg sodium

SNACK:
Nachos Deluxe
› **492** calories
› **16** g fat
    (**6** g saturated)
› **1,170** mg sodium

CHILDREN'S MEAL:
Chicken Nuggets
(4 pieces)
› **184** calories
› **10** g fat
    (**2** g saturated)
› **392** mg sodium

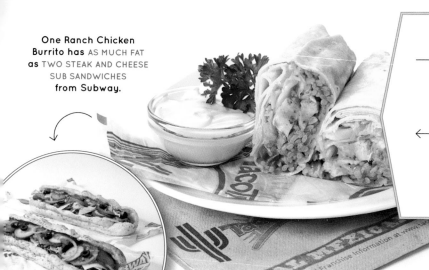

One Ranch Chicken Burrito has AS MUCH FAT as TWO STEAK AND CHEESE SUB SANDWICHES from Subway.

LOSE IT

RANCH CHICKEN BURRITO

507 CALORIES
19 G FAT (**4** G SATURATED)
1,356 MG SODIUM
62 G CARBOHYDRATES

TACO TIME

Why lose it? The rice and ranch dressing account for the extra calories and fat. The tortilla provides enough carbs, so you don't need the rice.

ALSO LOSE

BURRITO:
Beef & Cheese Burrito
› **556** calories
› **25** g fat
  (**11** g saturated)
› **1,430** mg sodium

SNACK:
Deluxe Mexi-Fries
(large)
› **674** calories
› **38** g fat
  (**12** g saturated)
› **1,949** mg sodium

CHILDREN'S MEAL:
Cheese Quesadilla
› **374** calories
› **18** g fat
  (**10** g saturated)
› **719** mg sodium

FOOD FACT

Getting the vocabulary right in a Mexican restaurant means a lot. A burrito is a stuffed, rolled, flour tortilla cooked on a griddle. A chimichanga is a deep-fried burrito with a savoury or sweet filling. A quesadilla is a flour tortilla filled with a combination of cheese, cooked meat and beans, folded in half and toasted or fried. A taco is a tortilla folded around a filling of meat and or cheese. A crisp tortilla is deep fried.

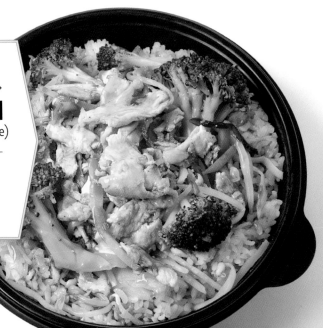

CHOOSE IT

→

CHICKEN TERIYAKI
(including white rice, pan-Asian sauce)

←

542 CALORIES
6 G FAT (**1** G SATURATED)
1,076 MG SODIUM
99 G CARBOHYDRATES

TERIYAKI EXPERIENCE

Teriyaki Experience/Made in Japan was established in 1986 in Toronto, with the goal of extending the traditional food court offerings. There are now over 100 Teriyaki Experience locations worldwide and right across Canada in shopping mall food courts, street fronts, universities, hospitals and theme parks. Vegetables and proteins are stir-fried in seconds and served over yakisoba noodles or steamed rice and a choice of sauces. The more health conscious can have meals cooked with water rather than oil.

Why choose it? The chicken is one of the lowest calorie and fat options for the teriyaki dishes, as the pan-Asian sauce is of the sauces. This dish has about a quarter of the fat of the Tofu Teriyaki. One ounce (28 g) of white chicken breast has 31 calories and 0.3 g fat; 1 oz (28 g) of firm tofu is 41 calories and 3 g fat.

→

ALSO CHOOSE

SOUP BOWL:
Shrimp Spicy Udon Noodle
› **286** calories
› **2** g fat
  (**0.3** g saturated)
› **1,944** mg sodium
› **48** g carbohydrates

VEGETARIAN:
Vegetable Pan-Asian Noodles
(including pan-Asian sauce)
› **213** calories
› **2** g fat
  (**0.3** g saturated)
› **36** mg sodium
› **41** g carbohydrates

SIDES:
Udon Noodles
› **158** calories
› **0** g fat
› **12** mg sodium
› **34** g carbohydrates

↓

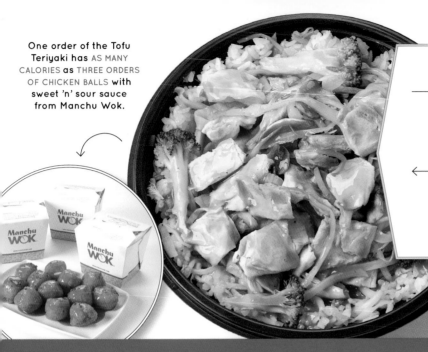

One order of the Tofu Teriyaki has AS MANY CALORIES as THREE ORDERS OF CHICKEN BALLS with sweet 'n' sour sauce from Manchu Wok.

LOSE IT

TOFU TERIYAKI
(including white rice, Hot and Spicy sauce)

918 CALORIES
25 G FAT (**3** G SATURATED)
1,520 MG SODIUM
119 G CARBOHYDRATES

TERIYAKI EXPERIENCE

Why lose it? It's interesting that of all the teriyakis on the menu the tofu (even without the sauce), has the most calories and fat, even though tofu is a vegetarian source of protein. The Hot and Spicy Sauce also has the most calories and fat of all the sauces.

ALSO LOSE

SOUP BOWL:
Tofu Yakisoba Noodle
› **466** calories
› **9** g fat
  (**1** g saturated)
› **1,749** mg sodium
› **72** g carbohydrates

VEGETARIAN:
Vegetable Teriyaki
(including Hot & Spicy Sauce, Asian cooking sauce)
› **664** calories
› **12**g fat
  (**3** g saturated)
› **1231** mg sodium
› **107** g carbohydrates

SIDES:
Yakisoba Noodles
› **267** calories
› **2** g fat
  (**0** g saturated)
› **71** mg sodium
› **52** g carbohydrates

HEALTH WARNING

When looking at the nutritionals of a restaurant serving tofu, you may notice that the tofu meal has more calories and fat than a chicken or beef dish. This is often due to the tofu being fried, which you may not even notice when it's buried in the rest of the meal. Four ounces (113 g) of fried tofu has 308 calories and 23 g of fat. Four ounces of grilled tofu has only 164 calories and 10 g of fat. By comparison, 4 ounces of ground beef has 310 calories and 20 g of fat.

CHOOSE IT →

HONEY DIP YEAST DONUT

210 CALORIES
8 G FAT (**3** G SATURATED)
11 G SUGAR

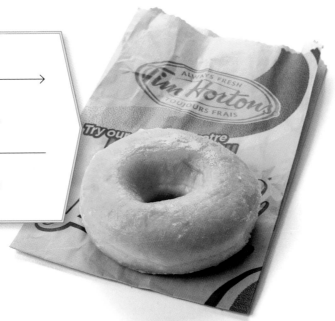

PART 1 TIM HORTONS

Tim Hortons was established in 1964 in Hamilton, Ontario, by Canadian hockey player Tim Horton and his business partner, Jim Charade. After Tim Horton died in a car crash in 1974, Ron Joyce made the chain into a multi-million-dollar franchise. The largest quick-service restaurant in Canada, Tim Hortons expanded from its original donut offerings into a wide selection of fresh coffee, baked goods, breakfasts and homestyle lunches. It is now bigger than McDonald's in Canada and has expanded to 3,040 stores

continued on page 150

Why choose it? The yeast variety of donut is lighter in texture due to the rising action of the yeast, and it has 110 fewer calories and less than half the fat, saturated fat and sugar than the Old-Fashioned Glazed Donut.

ALSO CHOOSE

BAGEL:
Cheddar Cheese Bagel
(including butter)
› **290** calories
› **11** g fat
   (**6** g saturated)
› **495** mg sodium

COFFEE:
Regular Coffee
(large, 18 oz/511 mL, including one cream, one milk, one sugar)
› **170** calories
› **8** g fat
   (**5** g saturated)
› **20** g sugar
› **20** g carbohydrates

BREAKFAST SANDWICH:
English Muffin
(including bacon, egg, cheese)
› **330** calories
› **15** g fat
   (**6** g saturated)
› **770** mg sodium

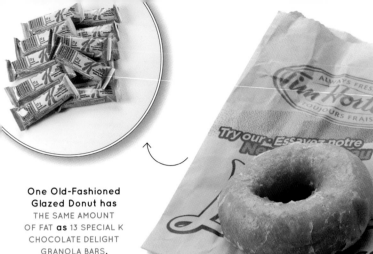

One Old-Fashioned
Glazed Donut has
THE SAME AMOUNT
OF FAT **as** 13 SPECIAL K
CHOCOLATE DELIGHT
GRANOLA BARS.

TIM HORTONS PART 1

Why lose it? This variety of donut, made without yeast, tends to be more cake-like and dense, resulting in a higher calorie, fat and sugar content. One donut has about 5 tsp (25 mL) of sugar.

TRIVIA

» The term "Double Double," which customers use at Tim Hortons to order a coffee with two creams and two sugars was added to the Oxford Canadian Dictionary in 2004.

» In 1964, a cup of coffee and a donut at Tim Hortons cost 10 cents.

» The busiest Tim Hortons is in Yellowknife, Northwest Territories.

ALSO LOSE

BAGEL:
12-Grain Bagel
(including plain cream cheese)
› **670** calories
› **23** g fat
   (**10** g saturated)
› **760** mg sodium

COFFEE:
Double Double
(large, 18 oz/511 mL, including two creams, two sugars)
› **270** calories
› **14** g fat
   (**9** g saturated)
› **30** g sugar
› **30** g carbohydrates

BREAKFAST SANDWICH:
Plain Bagel
(including sausage, egg, cheese)
› **550** calories
› **25** g fat
   (**10** g saturated)
› **1,160** mg sodium

CHOOSE IT

→

TOASTED CHICKEN CLUB
(including homestyle soft bun)

←

380 CALORIES
7 G FAT (**2** G SATURATED)
1,040 MG SODIUM

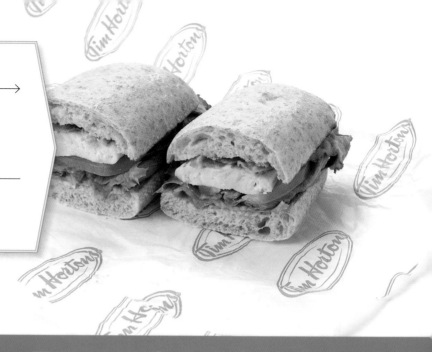

PART 2 TIM HORTONS

continued from page 148

nationwide, with 587 in the United States, Dubai and Abu Dhabi. The chain merged with Wendy's and recently co-branded with Cold Stone Creamery. The two most popular baked items, the Apple Fritter and the Dutchie, are as popular today as they were in the 1960s. Tim Hortons has a helpful nutritional chart and calculator available online, and it's easy to make healthy substitutions in the store, such using milk instead of cream in the Double Double.

Why choose it? Chicken is a better source of lean protein than the excess bacon in the BLT, and the mustard sauce is lighter than mayo, saving you more than half the fat and saturated fat. There's a small amount of bacon in this club.

ALSO CHOOSE

ICED CAPPUCCINO:
Iced Capp Original
(small, 10 oz/284 mL, including chocolate milk)
› **160** calories
› **0.5** g fat
 (**0.4** g saturated)
› **36** g sugar
› **36** g carbohydrates

SWEET BAKED GOOD:
Plain Croissant
› **270** calories
› **14** g fat
 (**6** g saturated)
› **4** g sugar
› **31** g carbohydrates

ICED COFFEE:
Mocha Iced Coffee
(large, 18 oz/511 mL, including milk)
› **240** calories
› **2** g fat
 (**1** g saturated)
› **31** g sugar
› **50** g carbohydrates

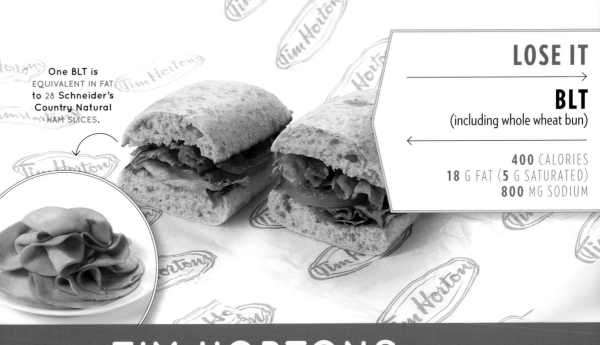

One BLT is EQUIVALENT IN FAT to 28 Schneider's Country Natural HAM SLICES.

LOSE IT

BLT
(including whole wheat bun)

400 CALORIES
18 G FAT (**5** G SATURATED)
800 MG SODIUM

TIM HORTONS PART 2

Why lose it? The extra bacon and light mayo is the main reason for the extra calories, and double the fat and saturated fat. Still, it's not a bad choice for lunch, but not a good source of protein.

ALSO LOSE

ICED CAPPUCCINO:
Iced Capp Supreme
(small, 10 oz/284 mL, including cream and hazelnut flavour)
› **320** calories
› **15** g fat
   (**10** g saturated)
› **40** g sugar
› **43** g carbohydrates

SWEET BAKED GOOD:
Date & Nut Muffin
› **430** calories
› **17** g fat
   (**2** g saturated)
› **35** g sugar
› **66** g carbohydrates

ICED COFFEE:
Mocha Iced Coffee
(large, 18 oz/511 mL, including cream)
› **330** calories
› **12** g fat
   (**7** g saturated)
› **31** g sugar
› **50** g carbohydrates

HOME COOKING

If you love bacon, there's a healthier and less fatty way to cook it than frying. You can actually bake your bacon. Line a pan with foil and set a rack overtop, so the bacon doesn't sit in the fat. Place the bacon in a single layer and bake for about 20 minutes or until it's as crispy as you like it. Place the bacon on paper towels to soak up the fat. No flipping required!

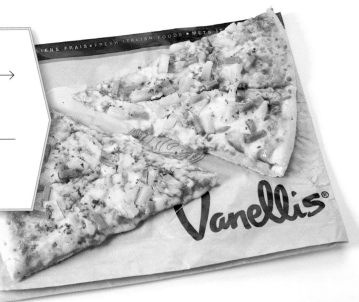

CHOOSE IT →

HAWAIIAN PIZZA
(2 slices)

←

860 CALORIES
26 G FAT (**12** G SATURATED)
2,580 MG SODIUM

Vanellis®

VANELLIS

Mrs. Vanelli's, now known as Vanellis, has been serving Canadians fresh, traditional Italian food since 1981. Today, Vanellis has 110 locations nationally and internationally, including in the United Arab Emirates and Saudi Arabia. With a variety of pizzas and pastas, Vanellis' emphasis is on fresh, healthy, quality food. The average slice of pizza has around 450 calories, 17 g of fat and almost a day's worth of sodium at 1,200 mg. Vanellis is also known for its create-your-own pasta meals. There's excellent nutritional information on its website.

Why choose it? The Hawaiian Pizza comes in at close to 400 fewer calories and 40 g less fat than the Roasted Vegetable Pesto Pizza. Clearly a better choice.

→

ALSO CHOOSE

ENTRÉES:
Meat Lasagna
› **500** calories
› **21** g fat
  (**11** g saturated)
› **1,200** mg sodium

PASTA:
Spaghetti
(including marinara sauce)
› **400** calories
› **3** g fat
  (**0** g saturated)
› **581** mg sodium

SALAD:
Greek Salad
› **180** calories
› **12** g fat
  (**5** g saturated)
› **480** mg sodium

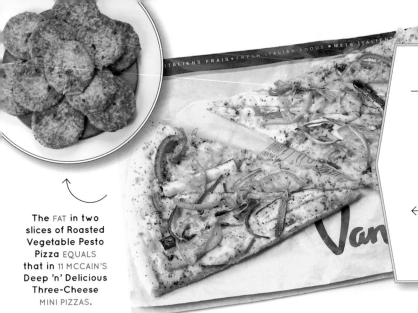

The FAT in two slices of Roasted Vegetable Pesto Pizza EQUALS that in 11 MCCAIN'S Deep 'n' Delicious Three-Cheese MINI PIZZAS.

ROASTED VEGETABLE PESTO PIZZA
(2 slices)

1,200 CALORIES
66 G FAT (**14** G SATURATED)
2,160 MG SODIUM

VANELLIS

Why lose it? This is a vegetarian pizza, but that doesn't mean it's lower in fat and calories. The garlic spread and pesto are oil based, adding up to three-quarters of a day's worth of calories, an entire day's worth of fat and over a day's worth of sodium.

FOOD FACT

Pesto is an Italian sauce originating in Genoa, in the northern part of the country. Traditionally, it is made with crushed garlic, basil, pine nuts, Parmesan cheese and olive oil, which is a healthy fat. But even healthy fats add up and must be eaten in moderation. One tablespoon (15 mL) has 80 calories and 7 g of fat. A usual serving of pesto in a pasta dish is close to 6 Tbsp (90 mL), which gives you 480 calories and 42 g of fat! You can cut the calories by substituting half the oil for water, chicken stock or light cream cheese.

ALSO LOSE

ENTRÉES:
Veal Cutlet
› **700** calories
› **32** g fat
  (**8** g saturated)
› **700** mg sodium

PASTA:
Cheese Tortellini
(including pesto)
› **780** calories
› **33** g fat
  (**7** g saturated)
› **790** mg sodium

SALAD:
Caesar Salad
› **520** calories
› **36** g fat
  (**8** g saturated)
› **5,000** mg sodium

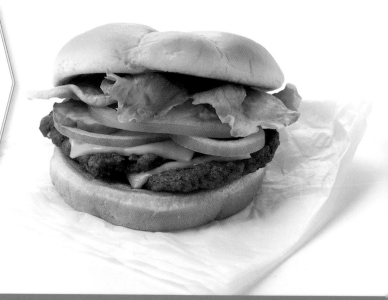

WENDY'S

Wendy's was founded in 1969 in Columbus, Ohio, by Dave Thomas, and today has about 6,650 locations internationally. It does not have a signature burger, but it differentiates itself by making its burger square instead of round. The children's menu has improved in recent years with more nutritious offerings, such as extra-lean deli-style sandwiches and yogurt with granola. Nutritionals are well described online with gluten free-meals and items under 510 calories and 10 grams of fat. Each item has an excellent description of what ingredients are in each meal.

Why choose it? With slightly less beef in the two junior patties and no cheese sauce, you save over 200 calories and 15 g of fat compared with the ½ lb double burger. Just ask for extra garnishes such as tomatoes, lettuce, pickles and onions to load up the sandwich.

→

ALSO CHOOSE

SALAD:
Apple Pecan Chicken Salad
(including pomegranate vinaigrette)
› **570** calories
› **29** g fat
  (**10** g saturated)
› **1,470** mg sodium

CHILDREN'S MEAL:
Chicken Nuggets
(4 pieces, including kids' fries, orange juice)
› **530** calories
› **20** g fat
  (**4** g saturated)
› **650** mg sodium

FROSTY:
Frosty Float with Vanilla Frosty & Coca-Cola
(small)
› **440** calories
› **9** g fat
  (**5** g saturated)
› **77** g sugar
› **80** g carbohydrates

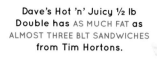

Dave's Hot 'n' Juicy ½ lb Double has AS MUCH FAT as ALMOST THREE BLT SANDWICHES from Tim Hortons.

DAVE'S HOT 'N' JUICY ½ LB DOUBLE

810 CALORIES
49 G FAT (**21** G SATURATED)
1,450 MG SODIUM

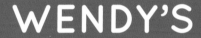

WENDY'S

Why lose it? The extra calories and fat comes from the two larger patties, cheese and cheese sauce and bacon and mayonnaise. This is half your daily calories, close to a day's worth of fat and a full day's worth of saturated fat.

HEALTH WARNING

Years ago, we set the upper limit of daily sodium intake at 2,500 mg, or about 1 tsp. Today we've cut that number to approximately 1,500 mg. That includes not just the salt we add in home cooking, that includes all the sodium in the many products and restaurant food consumed. The truth is that the average Canadian consumes about 4,500 mg of sodium a day! Excess sodium causes high blood pressure, which leads to heart disease and stroke. Eating less salt can cut cardiovascular disease by 25 percent.

ALSO LOSE

SALAD:
Baja Salad
(including creamy jalapeño dressing)
› **720** calories
› **46** g fat
  (**17** g saturated)
› **1,920** mg sodium

CHILDREN'S MEAL:
Jr. Cheeseburger Deluxe
(including kids' fries and J. Vanilla Frosty)
› **700** calories
› **29** g fat
  (**11** g saturated)
› **1,050** mg sodium

FROSTY:
Vanilla Bean Frosty Shake
(small, including whipped cream)
› **600** calories
› **13** g fat
  (**8** g saturated)
› **96** g sugar

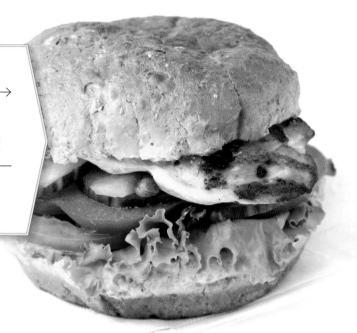

CHOOSE IT

MEDITERRANEAN CHICKEN BURGER

602 CALORIES
25 G FAT (**11** G SATURATED)
1,227 MG SODIUM

WHITE SPOT

White Spot first opened as a Vancouver drive-in in 1928. By the '50s, it was visited by 10,000 cars a day. Best known for its burgers, White Spot has served more full-service meals than any other casual dining brand in British Columbia. The décor consists of wood and rock elements with fireplaces, open kitchens and cozy booths. The menu includes Lifestyle Choices featuring the Heart and Stroke Foundation's Health Check seal. The nutritionals are online, but look carefully at the Modification tab to get an accurate total.

Why choose it? Grilled chicken is nothing more than chicken! With a small amount of cream cheese and a feta spread, and without any extra sauce such as aioli, this burger has almost 300 fewer calories and half the fat of the Portobello Provolone Veggie Burger.

ALSO CHOOSE

BREAKFAST:
Classic Eggs Benedict
(including hash browns)
› **678** calories
› **35** g fat
   (**14** g saturated)
› **1,737** mg sodium

ENTRÉE SALADS:
The Spot's Salad with Chargrilled Chicken
(including honey sherry dressing)
› **397** calories
› **24** g fat
   (**3** g saturated)
› **725** mg sodium

APPETIZER:
Chicken Dippers
(5 pieces, including plum sauce)
› **521** calories
› **18** g fat
   (**2** g saturated)
› **45** g carbohydrates
› **1,436** mg sodium

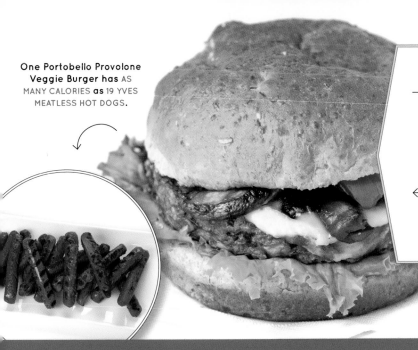

One Portobello Provolone Veggie Burger has AS MANY CALORIES as 19 YVES MEATLESS HOT DOGS.

PORTOBELLO PROVOLONE VEGGIE BURGER

889 CALORIES
50 G FAT (**13** G SATURATED)
1,332 MG SODIUM

WHITE SPOT

Why lose it? We would assume the veggie burger has to be better for us than a chicken burger. Nope! The calories and mega fats are hiding in the fillers—the provolone cheese and aioli.

ALSO LOSE

BREAKFAST:
Back Bacon, Cheddar & Mushroom Omelette
(including hash browns, toast)
› **1,261** calories
› **77** g fat
  (**21** g saturated)
› **1,723** mg sodium

ENTRÉE SALADS:
Santorini Chicken Salad
(including shallot dressing)
› **556** calories
› **37** g fat
  (**7** g saturated)
› **1,125** mg sodium

APPETIZER:
Sweet Potato Fries
(including chipotle mayo)
› **851** calories
› **55** g fat
  (**3** g saturated)
› **83** g carbohydrates
› **928** mg sodium

NUTRITION

We've been led to believe that veggie burgers are always a healthier option than beef or chicken burgers, and veggie burgers made from soy, beans or grains do have less fat and more fibre. An average veggie burger has about 3 g of total fat and 0.5 g of saturated fat versus a beef burger, which has 10 g of total fat and 3.5 g of saturated fat. But veggie burgers come pre-seasoned and have excess sodium—up to five times as much as a beef burger. They also contain less protein—5 to 15 g per veggie burger versus 11 g per meat burger—but are still considered a good source of protein overall.

ACKNOWLEDGEMENTS

Whitecap Books: Michael Burch, president – Thank you for bringing life to *Choose It and Lose It*. Your passion has made my work a joy. Michelle Furbacher, art director – your attention to detail was appreciated and made this book so precise and attractive. Lara Kordić, Theresa Best and Jesse Marchand, editors and proofreaders – for your excellent and essential work. Mauve Pagé, designer – the book looks incredible with your touch. Jeffrey Bryan and Debby de Groot, publicists – thank you for your work with respect to my many books with Whitecap. Nick Rundall, vice president and director of sales and marketing – thank you for a long and productive association.

Mike McColl, the fantastic photographer who brought out the best in every restaurant creation – truly a delight to work with.

Adrian Fiebig, photographer for my photo – somehow you seem to get the right angles every time.

Maureen Greenstein, make-up guru – thank you for your passion.

Barbara Cuden, my incredible assistant, who collected and analyzed the nutritional information for the restaurants. She also coordinated and assisted the photographer for the photo shoot. She's beyond diligent in her work and I couldn't work as effectively without her.

CityTV: Kevin Forget, Mohit Rajhans, Kate Moore, Tina Cortese and Jordan Schwartz – for believing in *Choose It and Lose It* and having me appear regularly on their shows.

National Post: Benjamin Errett and Maryam Siddiqi – for the opportunity to have a weekly *Choose It and Lose It* column.

Huffington Post: Jacqueline Delange and Ariana Huffington – for the opportunity to write bi-monthly health blogs.

ShareCare.com and Dr. Mehmet Oz – meeting Dr. Oz and being asked to write for his health website was a true honour. Thanks to Cathy Poley, who oversees my information.

Metro News: Dean Lisk and Izabela Szydlo – for the opportunity of writing a weekly *Choose It and Lose It* column and for now introducing weekly recipes.

680 News: Scott Metcalfe and John Hinnen – for the 12 weekly on-air *Food Bites* spots.

Dr. Harvey Skinner, Dean of Health at York University – for bringing me on as an adjunct professor to assist in what happens in and outside the world of the campus.

The Honorable Deb Matthews – for inviting me onto the Healthy Children's Task Force, to formulate recommendations for fighting childhood obesity.

Pickle Barrel restaurants: Peter Higley, chief executive officer – for giving me the opportunity to continually develop healthy recipes for the 12 restaurants in the chain as well as for Glow Fresh Grill and Glow Press. Stokely Wilson, executive chef – for recreating my healthy recipes for the consumer.

My wonderful household assistants: Lily Lim, Dang Idala and Mila Doloricon – for assisting me daily with my busy schedule.

INDEX

PRAISE FOR ROSE REISMAN

You can count on Rose Reisman to help you make smart choices when you eat out. In *Choose It and Lose It*, she dishes up the straight goods on great fast food and restaurant options. Spoiler alert: A salad is not always your best bet!

—IZABELA SZYDLO, food and family editor, *Metro News*

Rose is our go-to chef, with healthy recipes that are fun, simple and, most of all, delicious. *Choose It and Lose It* is a realistic approach to fast food and best choices.

—BEVERLY THOMSON, co-host, *Canada* AM

Rose Reisman is an inspiring woman with an intelligent voice. She has a unique drive for teaching people how to make healthy choices and for passing on her experience and the knowledge she has gained in the food industry. All of these qualities are represented in *Choose It and Lose It*. Mentor, leader and thought-provoker, Rose is a passionate advocate for healthy eating.

—SARAH THOMPSON, founder and publisher, *Women's Post*

Today, restaurant eating is a minefield of foods high in sugar, fat and salt, manufactured through taste to hook us into always wanting more while portion sizes have exploded. In *Choose It and Lose It*, Rose Reisman has created an expert guide to minimizing fast-food calories and controlling sugar, fat and salt intake. As a family physician, I can recommend this book as an invaluable tool for anyone wishing to navigate today's toxic fast-food restaurant environment.

—DAVID A. MACKLIN, MD, CCFP

In her new book, Rose Reisman shows why she is the best—she stays ahead of the trends and provides people with information that is ready-made for their busy lives. In *Choose It and Lose It*, she tackles restaurant dining, showing us how to navigate its caloric hazards in a no-nonsense way. Armed with this valuable information, we can make better, healthier choices. No simple task, but Rose makes it so easy.

—RON JOHNSON, editor, Post City Magazines